P9-DVQ-014

Treating Depression Effectively

OKANAGAN UNIVERSITY COLLEGE
LIBRARY
BRITISH COLUMBIA

Applying clinical guidelines

Sidney H Kennedy MD FRCPC
Professor of Psychiatry
University of Toronto
Psychiatrist-in-Chief
University Health Network
Toronto, Canada

Raymond W Lam MD FRCPC
Professor and Head
Division of Clinical Neuroscience
University of British Columbia
Vancouver, Canada

David J Nutt MD FRCP FRCPsych FMedSci
Professor of Psychopharmacology
University of Bristol
Bristol, UK

Michael E Thase MD
Professor of Psychiatry
University of Pittsburgh School of Medicine
Pittsburgh, PA, USA

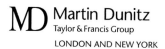
Martin Dunitz
Taylor & Francis Group
LONDON AND NEW YORK

© 2004 Martin Dunitz, an imprint of the Taylor & Francis Group plc

First published in the United Kingdom in 2004
by Martin Dunitz, an imprint of the Taylor & Francis Group plc, 11 New Fetter Lane,
London EC4P 4EE

Tel.:   +44 (0) 20 7583 9855
Fax.:   +44 (0) 20 7842 2298
E-mail: info@dunitz.co.uk
Website: http://www.dunitz.co.uk

All rights reserved. No part of this publication may be reproduced, stored in a retrieval
system, or transmitted, in any form or by any means, electronic, mechanical, photo-
copying, recording, or otherwise, without the prior permission of the publisher or in
accordance with the provisions of the Copyright, Designs and Patents Act 1988 or
under the terms of any licence permitting limited copying issued by the Copyright
Licensing Agency, 90 Tottenham Court Road, London W1P 0LP.

Although every effort has been made to ensure that all owners of copyright material
have been acknowledged in this publication, we would be glad to acknowledge in subsequent reprints or editions any omissions brought to our attention.

A CIP record for this book is available from the British Library.

ISBN 1-84184-328-8

Distributed in the USA by
Fulfilment Center
Taylor & Francis
10650 Toebben Drive
Independence, KY 41051, USA
Toll Free Tel.: +1 800 634 7064
E-mail: taylorandfrancis@thomsonlearning.com

Distributed in Canada by
Taylor & Francis
74 Rolark Drive
Scarborough, Ontario M1R 4G2, Canada
Toll Free Tel.: +1 877 226 2237
E-mail: tal_fran@istar.ca

Distributed in the rest of the world by
Thomson Publishing Services
Cheriton House
North Way
Andover, Hampshire SP10 5BE, UK
Tel.:   +44 (0)1264 332424
E-mail: salesorder.tandf@thomsonpublishingservices.co.uk

Printed and bound in Great Britain by The Cromwell Press Ltd, Trowbridge, Wilts.

Contents

About the authors

Sidney H Kennedy MD FRCPC
Professor of Psychiatry
University of Toronto
Psychiatrist-in-Chief
University Health Network
200 Elizabeth Street
Eaton North, 8th Floor, Room 222
Toronto, ON, M5G 2C4
Canada

Raymond W Lam MD FRCPC
Professor and Head
Division of Clinical Neuroscience
Department of Psychiatry
University of BC
2255 Wesbrook Mall
Vancouver, BC, V6T 2A1
Canada

David J Nutt FRCP FRCPsych FMedSci
Professor of Psychopharmacology
Dean of Clinical Medicine and Dentistry
Head of the Department of Clinical Medicine
University of Bristol
Psychopharmacology Unit
School of Medical Sciences
University Walk
Bristol BS8 1TD
United Kingdom

Michael E Thase MD
Department of Psychiatry
Thomas Detre Hall of the Western Psychiatric Institute and Clinic
University of Pittsburgh
3811 O'Hara Street
Pittsburgh, PA 15213
USA

Preface

This book grew out of a series of initiatives on depression guidelines by the Canadian Network for Mood and Anxiety Treatments (CANMAT, www.canmat.org). In 1999, *Guidelines for the Diagnosis and Pharmacological Treatment of Depression*[1] were developed primarily for use by family practitioners. Subsequently, in partnership with the Canadian Psychiatric Association, CANMAT published *Clinical Guidelines for the Treatment of Depressive Disorders*[2] for psychiatric specialist physicians in 2001. These guidelines were developed by the CANMAT Depression Work Group – Drs Murray Enns, Stanley Kutcher, Sagar Parikh, Arun Ravindran, Robin Reesal, Zindel Segal, Lillian Thorpe, Pierre Vincent and Diane Whitney – and chaired by Drs Sidney Kennedy and Raymond Lam.

We are very grateful to all our colleagues for their contributions to these earlier works and acknowledge the importance of their work as the foundation for this volume. We also appreciate the role of Ms Beata Eisfeld who provided editorial support throughout.

Sidney H Kennedy
Raymond W Lam
David J Nutt
Michael E Thase

---

1. CANMAT Depression Group. *Guidelines for the Diagnosis and Pharmacological Treatment of Depression*. Toronto, ON: Canadian Network for Mood and Anxiety Treatments, 1st edition, revised, 1999.

2. CANMAT Depression Work Group. Clinical guidelines for the treatment of depressive disorders. *Can J Psychiatry* 2001; **46**(Suppl 1): 1S–92S.

chapter 1

Prevalence, burden and diagnosis

Prevalence, course and burden of illness

Major depressive disorder (MDD) is among the most prevalent of medical illnesses. Recent epidemiological studies have highlighted the similarity in prevalence rates of depression in different countries (Figure 1.1). For many patients, depression is a chronic and recurrent illness. In follow-up studies, up to 30 percent of patients with MDD are still depressed after one year, 18 percent are ill after two years, and 12 percent remain ill after five years. Many patients treated for MDD still have residual and subsyndromal symptoms that result in poor outcomes, including higher risk for relapse and suicide, poor psychosocial function and higher mortality from other medical diseases. Among patients who recover from a depressive episode, over 50 percent will have a recurrence.

Given the high prevalence of depression, it is not surprising that the socioeconomic costs are also high. The World Health Organization (WHO), in a 1990 study comparing all medical illnesses, reported that depression was the fourth leading cause of health-related disability, and estimated that in 2020 depression would rank second only to heart disease as a worldwide cause of disability (Figure 1.2). The economic costs associated with premature mortality (e.g. from suicide), and the indirect costs such as reduced productivity and days off work, are staggering. People with depression are four times more likely to have days off work than people without depression (Figure 1.3). In the USA, the annual direct costs (hospitals, medications, doctor fees) of treating depression are estimated at US$12.4 billion. In the UK, excess mortality is estimated to cost over £4.7 million per year, while in Canada, the indirect cost of depression (lost productivity) is estimated at C$2.53 billion. Many nations now recognize that the diagnosis and treatment of depression are priorities for the medical system.

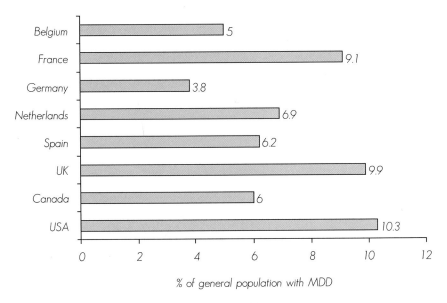

Figure 1.1 Six-month prevalence of MDD across different countries.

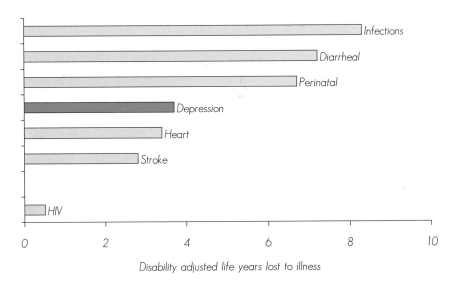

Figure 1.2 The Global Burden of Disease Study. In 1990, depression ranked fourth in disability.

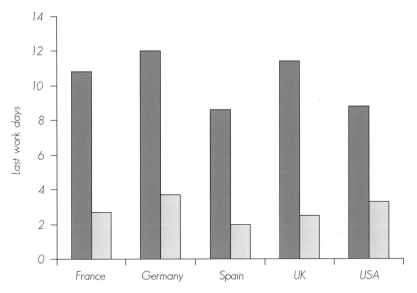

Figure 1.3 Lost work days in the last 6 months in depressed and non-depressed workers: ■, depressed; ☐, non-depressed.

Diagnosis of depression

The diagnostic criteria for an episode of MDD are similar in both DSM-IV-TR (Table 1.1) and ICD-10. Table 1.2 shows the differentiating features between MDD and normal bereavement. Despite the wide acceptance of these criteria, MDD is not well recognized or diagnosed in primary care settings because the presenting complaints are often physical in nature, such as pain, insomnia and fatigue. A comprehensive assessment of mood and physical symptoms in over 19 000 telephone respondents across Europe revealed a significant association between chronic painful physical symptoms and depression. The prevalence of MDD was over 10 percent in subjects with a chronic painful physical condition (CPPC) compared to 2.7 percent in subjects without a CPPC. Patients seen in primary care who present with unexplained physical symptoms should be screened for the presence of MDD (Table 1.3). While screening questionnaires can be used, a quick two-question screening for depression is helpful in these presentations:

1. In the last month, have you been bothered by little interest or pleasure in doing things?
2. In the last month, have you been feeling down, depressed or hopeless?

An answer of 'Yes' to either question should trigger a more detailed assessment.

Table 1.1 DSM-IV-TR Criteria for the diagnosis of Major Depressive Episode

A. Five (or more) of the following symptoms have been present during the same two-week period and represent a change from previous functioning; at least one of the symptoms is either (1) depressed mood or (2) loss of interest or pleasure:
   1. Depressed mood most of the day or nearly every day, as indicated by either subjective report (e.g. feels sad or empty) or observation made by others (e.g. appears tearful). Note: in children and adolescents, can be irritable mood.
   2. Markedly diminished interest or pleasure in all, or almost all, activities most of the day or nearly every day (as indicated by either subjective account or observation made by others).
   3. Significant weight loss when not dieting or weight gain (e.g. a change of more than 5 percent of body weight in a month), or decrease or increase in appetite nearly every day. Note: In children, consider failure to make expected weight gains.
   4. Insomnia or hypersomnia nearly every day.
   5. Psychomotor agitation or retardation nearly every day (observable by others; note merely subjective feelings of restlessness or being slowed down).
   6. Fatigue or loss of energy nearly every day.
   7. Feelings of worthlessness or excessive or inappropriate guilt (which may be delusional) nearly every day (not merely self-reproach or guilt about being sick).
   8. Diminished ability to think or concentrate, or indecisiveness, nearly every day (either by subjective account or as observed by others).
   9. Recurrent thoughts of death (not just fear of dying), recurrent suicidal ideation without a specific plan, or a suicide attempt or a specific plan for committing suicide.

B. The symptoms do not meet criteria for a Mixed Episode.
C. The symptoms cause clinically significant distress or impairment in social, occupational or other important areas of functioning.

Diagnostic instruments for clinical use

Semistructured clinical interviews can also help to confirm or validate a clinical diagnosis. For primary care physicians, the PRIME-MD interview takes approximately nine minutes to administer and has good predictive power for depression. For specialists, the Structured Clinical Interview for DSM-IV-TR (SCID) is the most widely used instrument but it requires training, is difficult to use and takes an hour or more to administer. The Mini International

Table 1.2 Features that help distinguish between bereavement and a Major Depressive Episode.

Feature	Bereavement	Major Depressive Episode
Time course	Less than two months	More than two months
Feelings of worthlessness	Absent	Present
Suicidal ideas	Absent	Common
Delusions of guilt, etc.	Absent	Possible
Psychomotor changes	Mild agitation	Marked slowing
Functional impairment	Mild	Marked to severe

Table 1.3 Patients with the following factors are at high risk for MDD and should be screened for depressive illness [Level 2]

- Chronic pain
- Chronic physical illness (diabetes, heart disease, etc.)
- Unexplained somatic symptoms
- Frequent visits
- Postpartum state
- Psychosocial stressor.

Neuropsychiatric Interview (MINI) is a more practical and convenient instrument and is available in a number of languages (free download available at www.medical-outcomes.com). The MINI takes 15–20 minutes to administer and aids in the diagnosis of 15 major psychiatric conditions in DSM-IV-TR and ICD-10.

A major diagnostic issue is differentiating between bipolar and unipolar depression. Hypomanic episodes, in particular, are difficult to identify in routine clinical practice. A scale such as the Mood Disorders Questionnaire may be a helpful tool to screen for bipolarity.

Subtypes of MDD

DSM-IV-TR includes a number of subtype specifiers for MDD based on cross-sectional clinical features or patterns of depressive episodes (Table 1.4). These various subtypes of MDD may have important implications for selection of treatment and, ultimately, prognosis (see Chapter 5). 'Anxious depression' is

Table 1.4 Specifiers of MDD according to DSM-IV-TR

Specifier	Key features
With melancholic features	Nonreactive mood, anhedonia, weight loss, guilt, psychomotor retardation or agitation, morning worsening of mood, early morning awakening
With atypical features	Reactive mood, oversleeping, overeating, leaden paralysis, interpersonal rejection sensitivity
With psychotic features	Hallucinations or delusions
With catatonic features	Catalepsy (waxy flexibility), catatonic excitement, negativism or mutism, mannerisms or stereotypies, echolalia or echopraxia. This subtype is not commonly seen in clinical practice
With chronic pattern	Two years or more with full criteria for MDE
With seasonal pattern	Regular onset and remission of depressive episodes during a particular season (usually fall/winter onset)
With postpartum onset	Onset of depressive episode within 4 weeks postpartum

not listed as a subtype within DSM-IV-TR but the term is often used to describe depressed patients who experience a preponderance of worry, tension and somatic symptoms related to anxiety. Symptoms of anxiety occur in 60–90 percent of patients with MDD and up to 50 percent of MDD patients may have a comorbid anxiety disorder (see Chapter 13).

Bibliography

Hirschfeld RM, Williams JB, Spitzer RL *et al*. Development and validation of a screening instrument for bipolar spectrum disorder: The Mood Disorder Questionnaire. *Am J Psychiatry* 2000; **157**: 1873–75.

Lepine JP, Gastpar M, Mendlewicz J, Tylee A. Depression in the community: the first pan-European study DEPRES (Depression Research in European Society). *Int Clin Psychopharmacol* 1997; **12**: 19–29.

Murray CJ, Lopez AD. Alternative projections of mortality and disability by cause 1990–2020: Global Burden of Disease Study. *Lancet* 1997; **349**: 1498–504.

Ohayon MM, Schatzberg AF. Using chronic pain to predict depressive morbidity in the general population. *Arch Gen Psychiatry* 2003; **60**: 39–47.

Parikh SV, Lam RW, CANMAT Depression Work Group. Clinical guidelines for the treatment of depressive disorders: I. Definitions, prevalence and health burden. *Can J Psychiatry* 2001; **46** (Suppl. 1): 13S–20S.

Spitzer RL, Williams JB, Kroenke K *et al*. Utility of a new procedure for diagnosing mental disorders in primary care. The PRIME-MD 1000 study. *JAMA* 1994; **272**: 1749–56.

Weissman MM, Bland RC, Canino GJ *et al*. Cross-national epidemiology of major depression and bipolar disorder. *JAMA* 1996; **276**: 293–9.

Chapter 2

Principles of management

Principles of management

The management of major depressive disorder (MDD) involves establishing a correct diagnosis and applying evidence-based and goal-directed principles of treatment. These treatment principles include recognizing and treating any co-existing medical conditions, building a therapeutic alliance with patients and choosing an appropriate treatment, as well as monitoring and maintaining response (Table 2.1).

Set goals of treatment

The overall goals of treatment are to achieve remission of symptoms, restore quality of life and prevent relapse or recurrence. The treatment of depression consists of two phases – acute and maintenance – each with specific goals,

Table 2.1 Nine principles of management for a major depressive episode

- Set clear goals for treatment
- Assess and treat comorbid medical conditions
- Assess suicide risk
- Establish a therapeutic alliance
- Consider psychotherapy
- Choose an appropriate antidepressant
- Enhance adherence (compliance) to treatment regimen
- Monitor treatment outcome
- Maintain response to treatment.

Table 2.2 The phases of treatment of depression

Phase	Duration	Objectives	Activities
Acute	6–12 weeks or longer	Remission of symptoms Return to previous full function	Establish therapeutic alliance Provide education Choose treatment Monitor response
Maintenance	6 months following remission, or longer	Prevention of relapse and recurrence	Provide education Manage side-effects Rehabilitation Monitor for recurrence

objectives and activities (Table 2.2). There is increasing recognition of the importance of achieving full remission of symptoms and return to baseline psychosocial function.

Treat comorbid medical conditions

Many medical conditions and medications are associated with symptoms of depression. It is important to recognize, investigate and treat comorbid conditions. Tables 2.3 and 2.4 show some general medical conditions and medications that are frequently associated with depression. However, depression can also co-exist with these conditions and requires independent treatment (see Chapter 13).

Assess suicide risk

Suicide risk should be regularly assessed throughout the course of treatment; when appropriate, family or friends should also be consulted. Paradoxically, suicide risk may increase when patients begin to show response, partly because improvement in energy level may precede improvement in mood.

Table 2.5 shows risk factors that are statistically correlated with suicide. One of the strongest clinical predictors is hopelessness, hence the assessment of suicide risk should include inquiries into the patient's plans or hopes. Table 2.6 shows the questions from the Mini International Neuropsychiatric Interview (MINI) to help assess suicide risk.

The management of suicidal thoughts can include distraction techniques (e.g. taking a walk or calling a friend), keeping a list of reasons for living, and access to telephone crisis lines. Involving the patient and significant others

Table 2.3 General medical conditions frequently associated with depression

Neurological disorders
  Alzheimer's disease
  Cerebrovascular disease
  Cerebral neoplasms
  Cerebral trauma
  CNS infections
  Dementia
  Epilepsy
  Extrapyramidal diseases
  Huntington's disease
  Hydrocephalus
  Migraine
  Multiple sclerosis
  Narcolepsy
  Parkinson's disease
  Progressive supranuclear palsy
  Sleep apnea
  Wilson's disease

Systemic disorders
  Viral and bacterial infections

Inflammatory disorders
  Rheumatoid arthritis
  Sjögren's syndrome
  Systemic lupus erythematosis
  Temporal arteritis

Endocrine disorders
  Adrenal
    Cushing's
    Addison's
    Hyperaldosteronism
  Menses related
  Parathyroid disorders
  Thyroid disorders
  Vitamin deficiencies
    B_{12}/Folate
    Vitamin C
    Niacin
    Thiamine

Other disorders
  Acquired immune deficiency syndrome (AIDS)
  Cancer
  Cardiopulmonary disease
  Klinefelter's syndrome
  Myocardial infarction
  Porphyrias
  Postoperative states
  Renal disease and uremia
  Systemic neoplasms

in the treatment plan is useful, as is documenting treatment plans. Patients who are at high suicide risk require urgent referral or hospitalization, which may include involuntary admission under local mental health laws.

Establish a therapeutic alliance

As with any treatment plan, informed consent should be obtained from the patient and/or the family. This provides an opportunity for education, which includes brief discussion of the causes of depression, its symptoms, options for treatments, risks and benefits of such treatments, possible side-effects and expectation of remission (Table 2.7). Primary care physicians are in a good position to establish a strong alliance as they already have a therapeutic

Table 2.4 Medications frequently associated with depression

Antibacterials and antifungal agents
Ampicillin
Clotrimazole
Cycloserine
Dapsone
Griseofulvin
Metronidazole
Nitrofurantoin
Sulfonamides
Streptomycin
Tetracycline
Thiocarbanilide

Cancer drugs
Beiomycin
C-Asparaginase
Mithramycin
Trimethoprim
Vincristine
Zidovudine

Cardiac and antihypertensive drugs
Beta-blockers
Clonidine
Digitalis
Guanethidine
Hydralazine
Lidocaine
Methyldopa
Prazosin
Reserpine
Procainamide

Analgesics and anti-inflammatory agents
Fenoprofen
Ibuprofen
Indomethacin
Opiates
Phenacetin
Phenylbutazone
Pentazocine

Stimulants and appetite suppressants
Amphetamine
Diethylpropion
Fenfluramine
Phenmetrazine

Sedatives and hypnotics
Barbiturates
Benzodiazepines
Chloral hydrate
Ethanol

Psychotropic medications
Antipsychotics

Neurological agents
Amatadine
Baclofen
Bromocriptine
Carbamazepine
Levodopa
Methosuximide
Phenytoin
Tetrabenazine

relationship with the patient from continuity of care. Through better understanding of the illness and its expected course, patients may have more trust in the proposed treatment plans. Patients may also feel more in control as they are actively involved in the decision-making process.

Consider psychotherapy

Psychotherapy is an effective treatment for depression in motivated patients. The evidence for efficacy is greatest for structured, time-limited

Table 2.4 *continued*

Steroids and hormones	Miscellaneous drugs
Corticosteroids	Acetazolamide
Danazol	Anticholinesterases
Oral contraceptives	Choline
Norethisterone	Cimetidine
Triamcinalone	Cyproheptadine
	Disulfiram
	Isotretinoin
	Meclizine
	Metaclopramide
	Methysergide
	Pizotifen
	Salbutamol

Table 2.5 Risk factors associated with suicide

Demographic	*Clinical*
Male	History and severity of prior attempts
Adolescent or geriatric age	Family history of depression and suicide
Unemployed	Hopeless
Socially isolated	Impulsive and agitated
Single/separated/divorced	Psychotic features
Poor support network	Alcohol and substance abuse
	Borderline/antisocial personality traits
	Chronic medical or psychiatric illnesses
	Recently discharged from hospital

psychotherapies, particularly cognitive behavioural therapy (CBT), inter-personal psychotherapy (IPT) and problem-solving therapy (PST, developed specifically for primary care) (Table 2.8). For MDD of mild to moderate severity, these psychotherapies are as efficacious as antidepressants and can be used as monotherapy (see Chapter 3). The Cognitive Behavioural Analysis System of Psychotherapy (CBASP) has been developed for use in chronic depression, with validation in a large clinical trial. Unfortunately, access to therapists who are trained in these evidence-based psychological treatments is limited in most countries.

Table 2.6 Suicidality assessment from the MINI

In the past month did you:			YES points
C1. Think that you would be better off dead or wish you were dead?	NO	YES	1
C2. Want to harm yourself?	NO	YES	2
C3. Think about suicide?	NO	YES	6
C4. Have a suicide plan?	NO	YES	10
C5. Attempt suicide?	NO	YES	10
In your lifetime:			
C6. Did you ever make a suicide attempt?	NO	YES	4

Add the total number of points for the answers (C1–C6) checked
YES and specify the level of suicide risk as follows   **TOTAL** _____

SUICIDE RISK - CURRENT

Low ☐	0-5 points	
Moderate ☐	6-9 points	
High ☐	10 or more points	

Adapted with permission from Sheehan *et al.* 1998.

Table 2.7 Suggested topics to be discussed before initiating treatment

- Depression is a medical disorder with serious consequences.
- The cause of depression is multifactorial, including biological/genetic factors ('chemical imbalance in the brain'; changes in neurotransmitters that are corrected by medications), psychological experiences, and social and economic stressors.
- Effective treatment is available with medications and/or psychotherapies.
- Adherence to treatment is important because the treatments take time.

Whether or not formal psychotherapy is offered, physicians should also provide supportive interventions that may improve patient outcomes (Table 2.9 and 2.10).

Choose an appropriate antidepressant

Antidepressants are often the treatment of choice for depression in primary care settings. A number are now available with different neurochemical actions and side-effect profiles. Most systematic reviews have not shown any clinically significant differences in standard response rates among antidepressants but

Table 2.8 Evidence-based psychotherapies for treatment of depression [Level 1]

Psychotherapy	General principles	Length of therapy
Cognitive Behavioural Therapy (CBT)	Identify automatic, maladaptive thoughts and distorted beliefs that lead to depressive moods Learn strategies to modify these beliefs and practice adaptive thinking patterns Use a systematic approach to reinforce positive coping behaviours	12 to 16 sessions
Interpersonal Therapy (IPT)	Identify significant interpersonal/relationship issues that led to, or arose from, depression (unresolved grief; role disputes; role transitions; social isolation) Focus on one or two of these issues, using problem-solving, dispute resolution and social skills training	12 to 16 sessions
Problem-Solving Therapy (PST)	Use a structured approach to identify and actively solve problems that contribute to depression	6 to 8 sessions
Cognitive Behavioural Analysis System of Psychotherapy (CBASP)	Use a combination of techniques from cognitive and interpersonal therapies to motivate patients with chronic depression to change their behaviours	16 to 20 sessions

Table 2.9 Simple and supportive interventions to manage depression [Level 3]

- Arrange regular follow-up visits
- Use the power of the prescription pad to 'prescribe' one brief walk per day and one pleasurable activity per day
- Keep a daily mood chart
- Recommend 'bibliotherapy' for depression, e.g. self-help workbooks: *The Feeling Good Handbook* by David D Burns (Plume Books, 1999); *Mind Over Mood* by Dennis Greenberger and Christine A Padesky (Zipper Books); the *Self-Care Depression Patient Guide* (available for free download at www.mheccu.ubc.ca)

Table 2.10 Helpful web resources for depression [Level 3]

• The Blue Pages (Australia)	www.bluepages.anu.edu.au
• Canadian Network for Mood and Anxiety Treatment	www.canmat.org
• MacArthur Foundation Initiative (Primary Care; USA)	www.primary-care.org
• Mental Health on the Internet (Canada)	www.mentalhealth.com
• National Institute of Mental Health (USA)	www.nimh.nih.gov
• PsychDirect (Canada)	www.psychdirect.com
• STAND (Stress, Anxiety and Depression; UK)	www.depression.org.uk

Table 2.11 Five simple messages to promote medication adherence [Level 2]

- Antidepressants are not addictive.
- Take your medication every day as prescribed.
- It may take two to four weeks to start noticing improvement.
- Do not stop medication without talking to your doctor, even if you are feeling better.
- Mild side-effects are common but are usually temporary. If you have more side-effects than you think reasonable, call your doctor.

there are some clinical factors that are important to consider when choosing a medication (see Chapters 4, 5 and 6).

Enhance treatment adherence

Adherence or compliance is crucial in the successful treatment of depression. Some simple messages to patients from their physicians have been shown to greatly enhance adherence to medication (Table 2.11).

Monitor treatment outcome

Patients should initially be followed on a weekly or bi-weekly basis until they achieve remission. Follow-up frequency can then be reduced to monthly or less often, depending on individual circumstances.

Most patients begin to respond to treatment within two to four weeks, show a good clinical response within six to eight weeks, and achieve full remission of symptoms by 8 to 12 weeks. Recovery of full baseline function to pre-depressed levels may take longer. If there is no response at all after four weeks of treatment, a change in the treatment plan is indicated (e.g. increasing the dose).

Response can be tracked using validated symptom rating scales. Traditionally, response is defined as a 50 percent or greater reduction in scores from baseline, while remission is defined as a score within the normal (not depressed) range. Decisions about strategies for non-response or inadequate response (see Chapter 9) are often based on degree of response as measured by severity scores.

There are many validated rating scales to assess severity of depression. The most widely used interviewer-rated scales include the Hamilton Depression Rating Scale (HDRS, various versions) and the Montgomery Asberg Depression Rating Scale (MADRS). One version of the HDRS includes items for so-called atypical symptoms of depression, such as overeating and over-sleeping; other abbreviated versions (e.g. the Ham-D–7, see Table 2.12) were developed for ease of administration by family physicians, psychiatrists and other health care specialists.

Patient-rated scales include the Beck Depression Inventory II (which includes items for atypical symptoms), the Hospital Anxiety and Depression Scale (HADS), and the Patient Health Questionnaire (PHQ), an easy-to-use, self-rated version of the PRIME-MD that is validated in primary care settings. Some of these measures are included in the Appendix, which starts on p. 21.

Maintenance response to treatment

For patients with a single episode of depression, the risk of relapse is two times higher in the first year following remission of symptoms than in the next year. Hence, once patients are in full remission from MDD, maintenance issues (e.g. how long should a patient continue to take their medication?) become important. Remission is an important target for both acute and maintenance phases as residual symptoms increase the relapse/recurrence rate, the degree of chronicity and suicide rate, and are associated with poor quality of life and greater health services utilization. Psychoeducation in the maintenance phase focuses on recognizing early signs of relapse or recurrence, and on adherence to medications. Practical aspects of maintenance therapy are summarized in Table 2.13.

Table 2.12 Seven-item Hamilton Rating Scale for Depression (Ham-D-7)

Please enter the appropriate score for each item

Item	Legend	Score
1. Depressed mood	0. Absent 1. These feelings indicated only on questioning 2. These feelings spontaneously reported verbally 3. Communicates feeling states non-verbally, i.e. through facial expression 4. Patient reports virtually only these feeling states in his or her spontaneous verbal and non-verbal communication	☐
2. Feelings of guilt	0. Absent 1. Self-reproach, feels he or she has let people down 2. Ideas of guilt or rumination over past errors or sinful deeds 3. Present illness is a punishment; delusions of guilt 4. Hears accusatory or denunciatory voices and/or experiences threatening visual hallucinations	☐
3. Work and activities	0. No difficulty 1. Thoughts and feelings of incapacity, fatigue or weakness related to activities, work or hobbies 2. Loss of interest in activities, hobbies or work, either directly reported by subject or indirect in listlessness, indecision and vacillation (feel has to push self to work or activities) 3. Decrease in actual time spent in activities or decrease in productivity. In hospital rate 3 if subject does not spend at least three hours a day in activities (hospital job or hobbies) exclusive of ward chores 4. Stopped working because of present illness. In hospital, rate if subject engages in no activities except ward chores, or if subject fails to perform ward chores unassisted	☐
4. Anxiety psychic	0. No difficulty 1. Subjective tension and irritability 2. Worrying about minor matters 3. Apprehensive attitude apparent in face or speech 4. Fears expressed without questioning	☐

Table 2.12 *continued*

Please enter the appropriate score for each item

Item	Legend	Score
5. Anxiety somatic	0. Absent 1. Mild 2. Moderate 3. Severe 4. Incapacitating	☐
6. Somatic symptoms (general)	0. None 1. Heaviness in limbs, back or head. Backaches, headache, muscle aches. Loss of energy and 'fatigability' 2. Any clear-cut symptoms rate 2	☐
7. Suicide	0. Absent 1. Feels life is not worth living 2. Wishes he or she were dead or any thoughts of possible death to self 3. Suicide ideas or gestures 4. Attempts at suicide (any serious attempt rates 4)	☐
	Total Score	☐☐

Score	Interpretation
0–3	Normal range; remission
4–7	Mild severity
8–15	Moderate severity
15 or higher	Marked/severe severity

Table 2.13 Recommendations for maintenance treatment of major depressive disorder

Recommendations	Evidence
All patients should continue on antidepressants for at least six months *after* a full remission of symptoms	Level 1
Patients with the following risk factors require longer maintenance treatment – at least two years, and for some, lifetime • Chronic episodes (> two years' duration) • Severe episodes (suicidality; psychotic depression) • Resistant or hard-to-treat episodes • Frequent episodes (two episodes in past two years) • Recurrent episodes (three or more lifetime episodes) • Older age (>65 years)	Level 2
The antidepressant dosage in the maintenance phase should be the same dosage as in the acute phase	Level 2
If the decision is made to discontinue an antidepressant, the antidepressant should be tapered slowly to avoid discontinuation symptoms	Level 3
Psychoeducation about early signs of relapse should continue (e.g. recurrence of sleep disturbances) and patients should have regular follow-up every two to three months	Level 3
Psychotherapy, e.g. cognitive behavioural therapy (CBT), may be helpful to prevent relapses	Level 2
Comorbid medical conditions and psychiatric disorders should be treated and rehabilitation programs (e.g. vocational counseling) may be helpful	Level 3

Appendix 2.A

Montgomery Asberg Depression Rating Scale (MADRS)

Note: Each item is scored on a 0 to 6 scale. Although the anchors list only even scores, odd numbers can be used if the rating is between scores.

	Response	Score
1. Apparent sadness Despondency, gloom and despair that is more than just ordinary transient low spirits	No sadness	0
	Looks dispirited but does brighten up without difficulty	2
	Appears sad and unhappy most of the time	4
	Looks miserable all the time; extremely despondent	6
2. Reported sadness Reports of depressed mood regardless of whether it is reflected in appearance or not. This includes low spirits, despondency or the feeling of being beyond help and without hope. Rate according to intensity duration and the extent to which the mood is reported to be influenced by events	Occasional sadness in keeping with the circumstances	0
	Sad or low but brightens up without difficulty	2
	Pervasive feelings of sadness or gloominess. The mood is still influenced by external circumstances	4
	Continuous or unvarying sadness, misery or despondency	6
3. Inner tension Feelings of ill-defined discomfort, edginess, inner turmoil, mental tension mounting to either panic, dread or anguish. Rate according to intensity frequency duration and the extent of reassurance called for	Placid with only fleeting inner tension	0
	Occasional feelings of edginess and ill-defined discomfort	2
	Continuous feelings of inner tension or intermittent panic which the patient can only master with some difficulty	4
	Unrelenting dread or anguish; overwhelming panic	6
4. Reduced sleep Reduced duration or depth of sleep compared to the subject's own normal pattern when well	Sleeps as usual	0
	Slight difficulty dropping off to sleep; slightly reduced light or fitful sleep	2
	Sleep reduced or broken by at least 2 hours	4
	Less than 2–3 hours of sleep	6
5. Reduced appetite Loss of appetite compared with when well. There may be a loss of desire for food or the need to force oneself to eat	Normal or increased appetite	0
	Slightly reduced appetite	2
	No appetites and food is tasteless	4
	Needs persuasion to eat at all	6

6. Concentration difficulties

Difficulties in collecting one's thoughts mounting to an incapacitating lack of concentration. This is rated according to the intensity frequency and degree of incapacity produced

No difficulties with concentrating	0
Occasional difficulties in collecting one's thoughts	2
Difficulties in concentrating and sustaining thought which reduces the ability to read or hold a conversation	4
Unable to read or converse without great difficulty	6

7. Lassitude

Difficulty in getting started; slowness in initiating and performing everyday activities

Hardly any difficulty in getting started; no sluggishness	0
Difficulties in starting activities	2
Difficulties in starting simple routine activities which are carried out with effort	4
Complete lassitude; unable to do anything without help	6

8. Inability to feel

Reduced interest in the surroundings or in activities that normally give pleasure. The ability to react with adequate emotion to circumstances is reduced

Normal interest in the surroundings and in other people	0
Reduced ability to enjoy usual interests	2
Loss of interest in the surroundings; loss of feelings for friends and acquaintances	4
Emotionally paralyzed; unable to feel anger grief or pleasure; complete or even painful failure to feel for close relatives and friends	6

9. Pessimistic thoughts

Feelings of guilt, inferiority, self-reproach, sinfulness remorse or ruin

None	0
Fluctuating ideas of failure, self-reproach or self-depreciation	2
Persistent self-accusation or definite but still rational ideas of guilt or sin; increasingly pessimistic about the future	4
Delusions of ruin, remorse or unredeemable sin; self-accusations which are absurd and unshakable	6

10. Suicidal thoughts

Feeling that life is not worth living and/or that a natural death would be welcome; presence of suicidal thoughts and the making of preparations for suicide

Enjoys life or takes it as it comes	0
Weary of life; only fleeting suicidal thoughts	2
Probably better off dead; suicidal thoughts common and suicide is considered as a possible solution but without specific plans or intentions	4
Explicit plans for suicide when there is an opportunity; active preparations for suicide	6

TOTAL SCORE

Score	Interpretation
0–11	Normal range; remission
12–19	Mild severity
20–29	Moderate severity
30 or higher	Marked/severe severity

Hospital Anxiety and Depression Scale (HADS)

Doctors are aware that emotions play an important part in most illnesses. If your doctor knows about these feelings he or she will be able to help you more. This questionnaire is designed to help your doctor to know how you feel. Read each item and place a firm tick in the box opposite the reply that comes closest to how you have been feeling in the past week. Don't take too long over your replies: your immediate reaction to each item will probably be more accurate than a long thought-out response.

Tick only one box in each section

1. I feel tense or wound up:
- ③ Most of the time ☐
- ② A lot of the time ☐
- ① Time to time ☐
- ⓪ Not at all ☐

2. I still enjoy the things I used to enjoy:
- ⓪ Definitely as much ☐
- ① Not quite so much ☐
- ② Only a little ☐
- ③ Hardly at all ☐

3. I get a sort of frightened feeling as if something awful is about to happen:
- ③ Very definitely and quite badly ☐
- ② Yes but not too badly ☐
- ① A little, but it doesn't worry me ☐
- ⓪ Not at all ☐

4. I can laugh and see the funny side of things:
- ⓪ As much as I always could ☐
- ① Not quite as much now ☐
- ② Definitely not so much now ☐
- ③ Not at all ☐

5. Worrying thoughts go through my mind:
- ③ A great deal of the time ☐
- ② A lot of the time ☐
- ① From time to time but not too often ☐
- ⓪ Only occasionally ☐

6. I feel cheerful:
- ③ Not at all ☐
- ② Not often ☐
- ① Sometimes ☐
- ⓪ Most of the time ☐

7. I can sit at ease and feel relaxed:
- ⓪ Definitely ☐
- ① Usually ☐
- ② Not often ☐
- ③ Not at all ☐

8. I feel as if I am slowed down:
- ③ Nearly all the time ☐
- ② Very often ☐
- ① Sometimes ☐
- ⓪ Not at all ☐

9. I get a sort of frightened feeling like butterflies in the stomach:
- ⓪ Not at all ☐
- ① Occasionally ☐
- ② Quite often ☐
- ③ Very often ☐

10. I have lost interest in my appearance:
- ③ Definitely ☐
- ② I don't take so much care as I should ☐
- ① I may not take quite as much care ☐
- ⓪ I take just as much care as ever ☐

11. I feel restless as if I have to be on the move:

③ Very much indeed ☐
② Quite a lot ☐
① Not very much ☐
⓪ Not at all ☐

12. I look forward with enjoyment to things:

⓪ As much as ever I did ☐
① Rather less than I used to ☐
② Definitely less than I used to ☐
③ Hardly at all ☐

13. I get sudden feelings of panic:

③ Very often indeed ☐
② Quite often ☐
① Not very often ☐
⓪ Not at all ☐

14. I can enjoy a good book or radio or TV program:

⓪ Often ☐
① Sometimes ☐
② Not often ☐
③ Very seldom ☐

Total for odd-numbered questions

Anxiety score:

Total for even-numbered questions

Depression score:

Scoring:
On either subscale a score of 8 or more is significant; a score of 11 or more is highly significant

Patient Health Questionnaire – PHQ-9
(www.primary-care.org)

1. Over the last 2 weeks, how often have you been bothered by any of the following problems?

	Not at all (0)	Several days (1)	More than half the days (2)	Nearly every day (3)
a. Little interest or pleasure in doing things	☐	☐	☐	☐
b. Feeling down, depressed or hopeless	☐	☐	☐	☐
c. Trouble falling/staying asleep; sleeping too much	☐	☐	☐	☐
d. Feeling tired or having little energy	☐	☐	☐	☐
e. Poor appetite or overeating	☐	☐	☐	☐
f. Feeling bad about yourself, or that you are a failure, or have let yourself or your family down	☐	☐	☐	☐
g. Trouble concentrating on things, such as reading the newspaper or watching TV	☐	☐	☐	☐
h. Moving or speaking so slowly that other people could have noticed. Or the opposite: being so fidgety or restless that you have been moving around more than usual	☐	☐	☐	☐
i. Thoughts that you would be better off dead or of hurting yourself in some way	☐	☐	☐	☐

2. If you checked off any problem on this questionnaire so far, how difficult have these problems made it for you to do your work, take care of things at home or get along with other people?

☐ Not difficult at all ☐ Somewhat difficult ☐ Very difficult ☐ Extremely difficult

TOTAL SCORE _____

Instructions: how to score the PHQ-9

Major depressive disorder is suggested if:

1. Of the nine items, five or more are checked as at least 'more than half the days'

2. Either item a. or b. is positive, that is, at least 'more than half the days'

Other depressive syndrome is suggested if:

1. Of the nine items, a. b. or c. are checked as at least 'more than half the days'
2. Either item a. or b. is positive, that is, at least 'more than half the days'.

Also, PHQ–9 scores can be used to plan and monitor treatment. To score the instrument, tally each response by the number value under the answer headings, (not at all = 0, several days = 1, more than half the days = 2 and nearly every day = 3). Add the numbers together to total the score on the bottom of the questionnaire. Interpret the score by using the guide below.

Guide for interpreting PHQ-9 scores

Score	Action
0-4	The score suggests the patient may not need depression treatment
5-14	Mild major depressive disorder. Physician uses clinical judgment about treatment, based on patient's duration of symptoms and functional impairment
15-19	Moderate-major depressive disorder. Warrants treatment for depression, using antidepressant, psychotherapy or a combination of treatment
20 or higher	Severe major depressive disorder. Warrants treatment with antidepressant, with or without psychotherapy, follow frequently.

Functional health assessment

The instrument also includes a functional health assessment. This asks the patient how emotional difficulties or problems impact work, things at home or relationships with other people. Patient responses can be one of four: Not difficult at all; Somewhat difficult; Very difficult; Extremely difficult. The last two responses suggest that the patient's functionality is impaired. After treatment begins, functional status and number score can be measured to assess patient improvement.

Bibliography

Beck AT, Steer RA, Ball R, Ranieri W. Comparison of Beck Depression Inventories -IA and -II in psychiatric outpatients. *J Pers Assess* 1996; **67**: 588–97.

Cummings JL. *Clinical Neuropsychiatry*. Orlando, Fl: Grune & Stratton, 1985.

Hamilton M. Development of a rating scale for primary depressive illness. *Br J Soc Clin Psych* 1967; **6**: 278–96.

Hirschfeld RM, Williams JB, Spitzer RL *et al*. Development and validation of a screening instrument for bipolar spectrum disorder: the Mood Disorder Questionnaire. *Am J Psychiatry* 2000; **157**: 1873–5.

Kroenke K, Spitzer RL, Williams JB. The PHQ–9: validity of a brief depression severity measure. *J Gen Intern Med* 2001; **16**: 606–13.

McIntyre R, Kennedy S, Bagby RM, Bakish D. Assessing full remission. *J Psychiatry Neurosci* 2002; **27**: 235–9.

Montgomery SA, Asberg M. A new depression scale designed to be sensitive to change. *Br J Psychiatry* 1979; **134**: 382–9.

Reesal RT, Lam RW, the CANMAT Depression Work Group. Clinical guidelines for the treatment of depressive disorders. II. Principles of management. *Can J Psychiatry* 2001; **46** (Suppl. 1): 21S–28S.

Sheehan DV, Lecrubier Y, Sheehan KH *et al*. The Mini-International Neuropsychiatric Interview (M.I.N.I.): the development and validation of a structured diagnostic psychiatric interview for DSM-IV and ICD–10. *J Clin Psychiatry* 1998; **59** (Suppl. 20): 22–33.

Spitzer RL, Williams JBW, Gibbon M, First MB. *Structured Clinical Interview for DSM-IV (SCID-IV)*. Washington DC: American Psychiatric Press, 1995.

Wilkinson MJ, Barczak P. Psychiatric screening in general practice: comparison of the general health questionnaire and the hospital anxiety depression scale. *J R Coll Gen Pract* 1988; **38**: 311–13.

Chapter 3

Psychotherapies, alone and in combination

Introduction

Psychotherapy is the oldest form of treatment for depression still in wide use, yet historically it has been the least well established in terms of evidence from controlled clinical trials. Once relegated to the sidelines of research on the differential therapeutics of mood disorders, several forms of depression-focused psychotherapy have now been identified as being efficacious treatments of major depressive disorder (MDD). These contemporary, depression-focused forms of therapy are characterized by a number of elements that have permitted investigation in controlled clinical trials: 1) they are intended to be shorter term, time-limited interventions (which approximate the length of the acute phase of pharmacotherapy); 2) they are conducted according to procedurally specified protocols; and 3) they are targeted to relieve the core symptoms of the depressive disorder.

The empirically verified forms of psychotherapy for depression have evolved from the disparate traditions of radical behaviorism, psychoanalysis and social work. Although each of these depression-focused psychotherapies emphasizes the importance of different aspects of the patient's phenomenological world, e.g. cognitive, behavioral or interpersonal factors that may be related to the onset or persistence of the depressive state, there are nevertheless a number of common or pan-theoretical elements. All emphasize pragmatic approaches to 'here and now' problems and a high level of activity on the part of the therapist. Monitoring of symptom outcomes is an integral part of treatment, and measures such as the Beck Depression Inventory are used routinely to document progress. The depression-focused psychotherapies also make ample use of psychoeducation, including both information about the nature of depression and how the methods of therapy will be used to address these problems. Many patients perceive these therapies to be directly relevant to their problems and experience an immediate morale-boosting effect, which serves to amplify expectations for success. Of course, the depression-focused psychotherapies also build upon a foundation of basic psychotherapeutic skills. These skills include the abilities to form an effective working alliance with the patient, maintain professional boundaries and promote a safe therapeutic milieu.

Treatment overview and limitations

The recommendations included in this chapter are based on the results of studies using specific forms of cognitive, behavioral and interpersonal psychotherapy. While evidence from randomized controlled trials (RCTs) is central to establishing treatment efficacy, it is noted that not all treatments have been evaluated in this manner. Moreover, the number of studies available to evaluate a particular treatment is not a reliable indicator of the intervention's inherent worth. Thus, the statement 'There is *no evidence* that Treatment X is effective' should not be viewed as synonymous with the statement that 'Treatment X is *not* effective.' Psychoanalytic psychotherapy, which has seldom been studied in controlled trials, represents a case in point. That said, an evidence-based approach to therapeutics gives higher rankings to interventions that have been evaluated in multiple RCTs and have been shown to have effects that surpass those of credible control groups (i.e. pill placebo or pseudotherapy conditions).

Depression-focused psychotherapy can be provided by clinical psychologists, psychiatrists and experienced masters degree prepared clinicians (e.g. social workers, nurses and counsellors). In our experience, virtually all capable therapists can learn to conduct at least one type of depression-focused psychotherapy. At least six months of supervised practice, augmented by readings and watching videotapes, is usually needed to achieve the minimum level of competence used to qualify therapists for participation in research studies. Some forms of therapy, such as Beck's model of cognitive therapy, may require an even longer period of training and supervision.

Although all forms of depression-focused psychotherapy have been adapted for use in group and couples formats, most research studies mirror practice patterns by continuing to emphasize individual models of treatment. Sessions typically last 45–60 minutes and are conducted either twice weekly or once a week. The latter is assuredly more common; the former may convey some advantage early in the course of treatment when working with more severely or chronically depressed patients. A standard course of therapy thus consists of 12 to 20 sessions provided across three to four months. Extended models of continuation (up to nine months) and maintenance (up to three years) phase psychotherapy have been developed for treatment of patients at high risk for relapse or recurrence.

It is noted that relatively few practitioners have received extensive training in one or more of these forms of therapy. Moreover, even fewer practicing clinicians actually employ 'pure' models of psychotherapy; most prefer to use an eclectic mix of interventions. If the specific techniques used in the different models of depression-focused psychotherapy actually contribute to treatment efficacy, eclecticism may run the risk of diluting the utility of therapy. In cognitive therapy, for example, several groups have found that routinely using an agenda to begin sessions and carefully attending to homework assignments correlate with better outcomes. As neither of these relatively basic strategies are particular favourites of a traditionally trained therapist, it is plausible that deviations from the 'pure' model of therapy may reduce efficacy. Therefore, the guidelines outlined below may not be applicable to the more widely practiced forms of psychotherapy.

Indications for psychotherapy alone

Several factors may be used to guide case selection for treatment with a depression-focused psychotherapy alone, instead of pharmacotherapy. First and foremost, the depression-focused psychotherapies have not been evaluated for treatment of the most severe depressive states, such as psychotic depression. Some evidence suggests that patients presenting with more severe forms of recurrent depression may be less likely to respond to psychotherapy alone (as compared with the combination of psychotherapy and pharmacotherapy). Similarly, psychotherapy alone should not be used to treat bipolar depression without appropriate concomitant pharmacotherapy. Case selection should therefore focus on ambulatory patients with mild-to-moderately severe nonpsychotic, nonbipolar depressive disorders. As is the case for other interventions, better outcomes are usually observed among people with more acute, circumscribed problems.

A second important factor is patient preference. Some people have decidedly nonmedical treatment preferences and feel more comfortable approaching their problems from a psychosocial perspective. Yet others have comparably strong negative biases against psychotherapy. When all other factors are equal, patients should be able to receive their treatment of first choice.

Availability of therapists is sometimes a rate-limiting step, particularly in rural areas. If a therapist is not trained in one of the newer, empirically validated therapies, factors such as communication with the referring physician, assessing syndromal outcome, and willingness to refer back for pharmacotherapy when the patient is not responding to treatment can serve as proxies for quality control.

General principles of cognitive, behavioural and interpersonal therapies

Many practitioners blend cognitive and behavioural therapies, the result being referred to as cognitive behaviour therapy (CBT). In the following brief descriptions, however, these models will be described separately for heuristic reasons.

Cognitive therapy

Beck's model of cognitive therapy (CT) is based on the proposition that changes in depressed patients' maladaptive ways of thinking are the most direct means to achieve durable symptomatic relief. CT is aimed at modifying three levels of cognition. At the most fundamental level are schema, which are the core beliefs or unspoken principles that organize perception and guide behaviour. The knowledge of how to tie a shoe lace is an example of a simple schema used in everyday life. Of greatest relevance to depression are schema about lovability, self-worth, fairness and the trustworthiness of significant others.

At a second, more accessible level are dysfunctional attitudes, which are the more specific rules that translate or operationalize schema. For example, someone with a schema of low self-worth may approach life with the following operational attitude: 'I must succeed at everything I do.' A depressogenic attributional style (i.e. the predisposition to view a negative event to have large, irreversible effects) is another example of this level of cognitive dysfunction.

At the most superficial level are the thoughts, images, memories and daydreams that comprise the depressed person's waking mental life. These various types of 'surface' cognition can be recorded as a way of objectifying a depressed individual's running negative commentary of about self, world and future (which was referred to by Beck as the 'cognitive triad'). When such spontaneous cognitions are associated with dysphoric effects, they are referred to as automatic negative thoughts. Turning one of Freud's dictums on its head, Beck asserted that affect is the 'royal road to cognition.' Cognitive therapists help patients to recognize the link between depressive feelings and habitual ways of thinking and begin to organize automatic negative thoughts into themes, which in turn can guide case formulations about schematic vulnerability.

The cognitive model of psychopathology also emphasizes the importance of information processing biases that tend to increase states of affective distress. These biases include processes such as selective abstraction, overgeneralization, emotional reasoning, all-or-none thinking, personalization and 'mind-reading'. During depressive states memory retrieval is biased, with relatively decreased access to positive or disconfirmatory memories and greater access to mood congruent, negatively themed memories.

Effective cognitive therapists employ a high degree of structure to help patients focus on learning more active and effective ways of coping. Each session is organized around an agenda that almost always includes three activities: symptom evaluation; review of homework; and selection of new homework activities. These tasks are sandwiched around two or three other segments of in-session work.

Therapists use a style of interaction referred to as collaborative empiricism, which emphasizes guided discovery (also known as Socratic questioning). The therapist's role as a guide or teacher is thus emphasized, although it should not be at the expense of maintaining an empathic rapport. Therapists seek explicit feedback at each transition point in a session to help ensure that patients are in 'synch' with the material being discussed, and feel understood by (and connected to) the therapist.

In a typical course of CT (Table 3.1), the early phase (e.g. sessions 1 to 6) emphasizes establishing a therapeutic relationship, enculturating patients to the style of the therapy, educating them about the cognitive model of treatment, identifying target symptoms and setting shorter-term goals, and establishing the relationship between depressive feelings and automatic negative thoughts. In practice, it is usually helpful to also use behavioural activation strategies (described below) to help patients begin to engage in more productive activities.

The middle phase of therapy (e.g. sessions 7 to 12) centers around extensive use of a systematized approach to addressing automatic negative

Table 3.1 Phases of treatment with CBT

Early phase (sessions 1 to 6)
- Establishes therapeutic relationship
- Identifies target symptoms and short-term goals
- Educates about model and clarifies links between depressive feelings and automatic negative thoughts

Middle phase (sessions 7 to 12)
- Systematized approach to addressing automatic negative thoughts – Daily Record of Dysfunctional Thoughts

Latter phase (session 13 to end)
- Identification of risk factors for relapse
- Implementation of balanced view of self, the world and the future
- Preparation for termination

thoughts. Using a form called the Daily Record of Dysfunctional Thoughts, patients learn to focus in on periods of low mood by recording the following sequence: the event; mood state (pre-intervention); automatic negative thoughts; rational alternatives; and mood state (postintervention). Asking patients to write down both their automatic negative thoughts as well as rational alternatives helps the individual to examine the basis for these and to consider different (less biased) interpretations.

The later phases of CT (e.g. sessions 12 through termination) address preparing the patient for termination, including identification of high-risk situations relevant to relapse risk and facilitating self-directed learning via more independent homework tasks. Longer-term goals are set and a life plan is developed to help guide goal attainment. Ideally, a successfully treated patient will have recognized their schematic vulnerability, practiced living with more functional attitudes, and have begun to implement a life plan that will support a more balanced way of thinking about oneself, the world around and the future.

In some regions it may be difficult to find a capable, well-trained cognitive therapist. It may be helpful to contact The Academy for Cognitive Therapy (*www.academyofct.org*) to obtain a referral. The shortage of trained therapists may be offset in the future by the use of computer-assisted models of CT, such as the one developed for CD-ROM by Wright, Wright and Beck. A number of useful self-help manuals are also available, including *Mind over Mood* (Greenberger and Padesky 1995) and *The Feeling Good Handbook* (Burns 1999).

Behaviour therapy

Behaviour therapies (BTs) are based on the fact that depression is associated with decreased levels of operant (goal-directed) behaviour and a resulting deficit in positive reinforcement. The anhedonia of depression may actually reduce the reinforcing 'power' of pleasurable activities, underpinning cognitions such as 'Why bother – it won't make a difference.' Most depressed people also manifest behavioural excesses (i.e. crying, complaining and other signs of hyperarousal including anxiety and insomnia). A third set of targets for behavioural interventions results from recognition that some people prone to depression have longstanding difficulties in assertiveness, conflict resolution and problem solving. These social skill deficits increase the likelihood of difficulties in both intimate relationships and vocational pursuits.

In the early stages of behaviour therapy, patients learn to monitor their moods and activities and to rate the associated degree of mastery and pleasure. Typically, a patient would be asked to keep an hour-by-hour or day-by-day log of their activities and mood states. If this functional analysis reveals deficits in mastery or pleasure, homework assignments are used to increase the level of behavioural activation. Large, potentially overwhelming tasks are tackled by homework assignments that break down a complex chain of behaviours into more manageable units; this technique is referred to as graded task assignment. Specific behavioural strategies, including progressive deep muscle relaxation, diaphragmatic breathing, and thought stopping, are utilized when indicated to help patients cope with symptoms of anxiety and insomnia. Social skills training (including behavioural rehearsal and role playing) might be used later in the course of therapy to help increase self-confidence and address the patient's difficulties in relationships. Similarly, a step-wise approach to problem solving may be used to help patients incorporate a more systematic method into their repertoire to help lessen the impact of future stressors. The book *Coping with Depression* outlines a 12-session course of behaviour therapy developed for individual or group interventions.

Cognitive Behavioural Analysis System of Psychotherapy

A hybrid model of treatment, referred to as the Cognitive Behavioural Analysis System of Psychotherapy (CBASP), was developed by McCullough (2000) to address the more pervasive problems of patients with chronic forms of depression. CBASP is distinguished from CT by the use of a standardized, relationship-based approach to problem solving. This method builds upon a situational analysis of behaviour by incorporating the patient's desired outcomes and an appraisal of what prevented obtaining that desired outcome. In short, CBASP takes a very 'molecular', situation-by-situation approach to help patients learn to become more effective in their interpersonal relations.

Interpersonal psychotherapy

By contrast, interpersonal psychotherapy (IPT) uses more conventional 'talk therapy' strategies to address the problems that patients face in relation to the onset or persistence of the depressive disorder. There is a basic assumption in IPT that depression is a biopsychosocial phenomenon and that addressing interpersonal difficulties, whether they are contributing factors or consequences of the disorder, will facilitate symptomatic improvement. Paradoxically, IPT is the form of depression-focused psychotherapy that most explicitly embraces a medical or illness model, yet takes the most decidedly traditional approach to foster symptom resolution.

The work of IPT revolves around addressing problems in one or more of the following themes: unresolved grief; role transitions; role disputes; and interpersonal deficits (i.e. loneliness and social isolation). This therapy is less structured than CT or CBASP, although therapists may actively assist the patient to clarify, resolve and/or better cope with their interpersonal problems. Strategies include eliciting emotional expression to facilitate grief work, brainstorming to identify novel methods to resolve impasses in communication with significant others, acceptance of problems that can't be changed, and encouragement to try out different types of social activities to reduce social isolation.

IPT is typically conducted with 12–16 weekly sessions (Table 3.2), which can be viewed as divisible into three phases. Therapists use the earlier sessions to

---

Table 3.2 Phases of treatment with IPT

Early phase (sessions 1 to 6)
- Establish a working alliance
- Provide education about depression and the IPT model
- Develop interpersonal industry

Middle phase (sessions 7 to 12)
- Work on resolution of problem areas defined in early phase, e.g. facilitate grief work, resolve impasses in communication with significant others, etc.

Latter phase (sessions 13 to 16)
- Review course of treatment and suggest techniques to deal with anticipated future problems

develop the interpersonal inventory, as well as to establish a working alliance, provide education about depression and aclimatize patients to the workings of psychotherapy. The middle phase of IPT moves is intended for work on resolution of one or more of the problem areas noted on the interpersonal inventory.

Although IPT does not prescribe the use of specific cognitive or behavioural strategies or make regular use of formal homework assignments, there is a degree of technical eclecticism permitted that results in overlap with CT and BT. A final or termination phase (e.g. sessions 13–16) is devoted to reviewing the course of treatment and discussing anticipated future problems. One resource for learning more about IPT is the textbook *A Comprehensive Guide to Interpersonal Psychotherapy* (Weissman *et al.* 2000).

Effectiveness of depression-focused psychotherapies

As of May 2003, there were nearly 100 published studies that evaluate the efficacy of one or more forms of depression-focused psychotherapy. The most clear-cut evidence comes from studies that have used waiting lists or pseudotherapy control conditions. A number of meta-analyses document that cognitive and behavioural therapies have definite efficacy when compared with these relatively weak standards. Although only two IPT studies used such a low contact control condition, both studies documented significant antidepressant effects. For psychiatrists, RCTs that compare a depression-focused psychotherapy with antidepressant pharmacotherapy provide a more meaningful index of therapeutic benefit. Again, meta-analyses document efficacy – all three forms of depression-focused psychotherapy have effects that are comparable (definitely *not inferior*) to those documented for antidepressants as administered in these trials. However, only a few RCTs have employed a placebo control group to help confirm that the antidepressant was indeed effective and those that did have yielded mixed results.

Although the weight of the evidence from published RCTs favours CT, there is little evidence that one model of depression-focused therapy is more effective than any other. This is particularly true after the impact of the allegiance of the studies' principal investigators is taken into account.

Only two trials have directly compared CT and IPT. The results of the first of these studies, the Treatment of Depression Collaborative Research Project (TDCRP), have had the most impact. This trial was relatively large (i.e. 250 patients), had the imprimatur of the US Government's National Institute of Mental Health, and exemplified the state of the art in psychotherapy outcome research at the time the study was conducted (1981–84). Moreover, in addition to using an active control group, treatment with the antidepressant imipramine, the study included a fourth group that received double-blind placebo. Overall, the TDCRP found some advantage for each of the active treatments when compared to the placebo control group, but the differences were modest and inconsistent. Among the less severely depressed subgroup of patients (~60% of the sample), the patients treated with placebo generally did as well as those who received the active treatments. In the more severely symptomatic subgroup, imipramine therapy was definitely superior to placebo, with IPT and CT showing intermediate effects. Comparing the two psychotherapies, nonsignificant trends favoured IPT over CT, and there was some evidence of differential predictors of psychotherapy response. Within the IPT cell, therapy was more effective among patients with endogenous features, less pathologic personality profiles and less social impairment. Among those treated with CT, outcomes were better for married patients, as well as those with atypical depression or relatively low levels of cognitive distortions. A strong therapeutic alliance was predictive of improvement in all four treatment modalities, whereas chronicity of illness predicted poorer across-the-board outcomes.

The second trial compared response to IPT and CBT among a predominantly male, HIV positive patient group with either dysthymia or MDD. In this 16-week trial, IPT (n = 24) and supportive therapy plus imipramine (n = 26) were comparably effective and both interventions were significantly more effective than both CT (n = 27) and supportive therapy alone. Comparing the two psychotherapies, the outcome of the IPT group was strikingly superior to that of the CT group (e.g. a mean difference in final HAM-D scores of nearly 0.8 standard deviation units).

Although a number of studies have compared CT and BT, most studies were inconclusive because of low statistical power and, frankly, flawed by strong investigator allegiance effects. One more recent, large (n = 150) study found CT, BT and their combination to be comparably effective treatments for outpatients with mild-to-moderately severe depressive episodes.

A small number of studies have contrasted group and individual forms of CT or BT. Results of meta-analyses of comparative studies documented that group forms of CBT were effective (compared to waiting list controls), with antidepressant effects that approached the magnitude of individual therapy. Likewise, BT and CT have been modified for treatment of depression within a couple's format. Among depressed patients with distressed marriages, the couples approach had antidepressant effects comparable to individual CT, with broader, mode-specific effects on dyadic adjustment. This information is summarized in Table 3.3.

Table 3.3 Recommendations for individual, group and marital therapies

Therapeutic choice	Recommendations	Evidence
First	Individual CBT or IPT for nonpsychotic nonbipolar MDD	Level 1
Second	Group formats of CBT	Level 2
	There is less evidence for efficacy of group as compared to individual forms of psychotherapy and the latter is recommended for treatment of more severe depressive episodes	
Third	Marital or couples therapy, in patients with significant marital distress	Level 2

Other psychosocial treatments for depression

The simplest, least expensive approach to treatment is bibliotherapy (Table 3.4), which relies upon books such as *The Feeling Good Handbook* (Burns 1999) to convey the therapeutic intervention. Six studies have compared bibliotherapy to a waiting list control condition in milder depressive states. A meta-analysis of these studies concluded that bibliotherapy has a definite therapeutic effect, which may be especially useful for depressed people who are unable to see a psychotherapist. Several small studies have found that computerized applications of CT likewise have antidepressant effects that surpass the improvements observed in waiting list control conditions.

Yoga and meditation may facilitate self-awareness, acceptance and tolerance of affective experience, which are useful skills for dealing with some aspects of depression, such as anxious hyperarousal and ruminative negative thinking. However, there are no well-controlled RCTs of these approaches.

Table 3.4 Recommendations for other psychosocial treatments

Therapeutic choice	Recommendations	Evidence
First	None are recommended in lieu of standard treatments	Level 1
	Exercise is an effective adjunct to standard treatments	
Second	Bibliotherapy – this should be considered an adjunct treatment to other first line treatments	Level 2
Third	Yoga – this should be considered an adjunct treatment to other first line treatments	Level 3

By contrast, aerobic exercise has been studied and found to have antidepressant effects of sufficient magnitude to warrant use as a routine adjunct to standard therapies.

Preventive effects of depression-focused psychotherapies

The relatively higher shorter-term costs of the depression-focused psychotherapies could be offset if it was shown that treatment had enduring effects on subsyndromal, residual symptoms or relapse rates. This is particularly important because the well-established preventive effects of pharmacotherapy are essentially lost within six months of stopping antidepressants.

Some evidence of durability of antidepressant effects following acute phase CT has been reported. In four of the smaller RCTs follow-up studies of patients were conducted for up to 24 months after CT and pharmacotherapy were discontinued. In these studies, patients who had responded to pharmacotherapy had a higher probability of relapse after withdrawal of medication than patients who had responded to CT (e.g. 50–66% relapse risk following medication discontinuation versus 20% following termination of CT). However, this difference was not apparent in the TDCRP, although it should be recalled that CT was not a particularly effective treatment in that study. No evidence of enduring antidepressant effects was observed for IPT in either the TDCRP or the initial RCT conducted by the treatment's developers.

Work by Thase, Jarrett and their colleagues suggests that an enduring benefit following a time-limited course of CT is contingent upon achieving a full and stable remission within the first eight weeks of therapy. When response was so classified, fewer than 10% of this 'good prognosis' group relapsed across one year after treatment termination, as compared to 50–60% of those who responded in a slower or less complete manner.

Continuation phase psychotherapy

Jarrett and colleagues subsequently developed a ten-session model continuation phase CT and tested its preventive efficacy across the first eight months after termination of acute phase therapy. The efficacy of this strategy was suggested in a case control study and confirmed (relative to an assessment-only control condition) in a prospective RCT. Of note, patients who remitted rapidly and fully obtained no further benefit from continuation phase

Table 3.5 Recommendations for psychotherapy as maintenance treatment

Recommendations	Evidence
• There is limited evidence to recommend psychotherapy as maintenance treatment	Level 2
• Acute phase treatment with CT may have sustained benefits that provide modest protection against relapse	Level 2
• Longer-term models of CT and IPT may reduce relapse rates, although there is insufficient evidence about the optimal frequency and duration of maintenance sessions	Level 2

therapy – their low risk could not be reduced further. For the patients whose response to CT was slower or less complete, by contrast, continuation phase therapy conveyed a three-fold reduction in relapse risk.

Maintenance phase models of psychotherapies have been developed as an analog to prophylactic pharmacotherapy (Table 3.5). Two studies have investigated the impact of monthly sessions of IPT after successful acute phase treatment in combination with imipramine. In the first study of adults with a history of highly recurrent depressive episodes, monthly sessions of IPT resulted in a modest reduction in recurrence risk after withdrawal of pharmacotherapy. However, maintenance IPT did not significantly extend survival time for patients who continued to take imipramine and the effect of IPT alone paled in comparison with the preventive effect of imipramine. In the second study, which focused on recurrent depression in late life, the effects of IPT and nortriptyline were both modest when compared with maintenance therapy with the combination.

Combining antidepressants and psychotherapy

For many years, combined treatment was one of the cornerstones of the practice of psychiatry. However, the additional costs of combined treatment (not only economic costs but also costs associated with side-effects and time for treatment) may not be justified if results are not clearly superior to monotherapies. Unfortunately, there are very few adequately powered studies evaluating combined treatment. There are three key reasons to consider combining psychotherapy and pharmacotherapy (Table 3.6): 1) increasing acute phase

Table 3.6 Recommendations for concurrent combined treatment

Acute phase treatment – concurrent combined treatment is recommended in the following circumstances:

Therapeutic choice	Recommendations	Evidence
First	Severe depression – IPT + pharmacotherapy are more effective than either treatment alone	Level 1
	Chronic depression – the combination of cognitive behavioural analysis system of psychotherapy (CBASP) and nefazodone is more effective than either treatment alone	Level 2

Maintenance phase treatment – concurrent combined treatment is recommended in the following circumstances:

Therapeutic choice	Recommendations	Evidence
First	Elderly patients – IPT + nortriptyline reduces recurrence rates compared to either treatment alone in patients treated with the combination in the acute phase	Level 2

efficacy; 2) broadening the scope of response; and 3) reducing the subsequent risk of relapse/recurrence. However, most of the earlier studies of combined treatment failed to detect additive effects on any of these indexes. This lack of effect was probably the result of a type 2 error because none of those studies had adequate statistical power to detect moderately sized additive effects. It is also plausible that it is not necessary to combine treatment modalities for the relatively easier-to-treat depressions, i.e. milder, more acute first or second episode without significant comorbidity.

The effectiveness of combined treatment was evaluated in a pooled analysis of 595 depressed outpatients who had received 16 weeks of CT, IPT alone or IPT plus antidepressants There was a modest difference in remission rates among the less severely depressed patients (psychotherapy alone, 37%; combined treatment, 48%). Moreover, combined treatment conveyed a marked advantage (over psychotherapy alone) for patients with more severe depressive episodes (remission rates: 49% versus 25%).

In a RCT enrolling 681 chronically depressed patients, the combination of nefazodone and CBASP was significantly more effective than either treatment alone (response rates for CBASP, nefazodone and the combination were 48%, 48% and 73%, respectively). The combination group benefited from the earlier temporal course of improvement resulting from pharmacotherapy as well as the later emerging benefit of the psychotherapy.

With a few exceptions, combined treatment is provided either by a psychiatrist or a physician and a nonmedical therapist working together. When two clinicians are involved, ongoing communication to lessen the impact of splitting, provision of coherent education about both modalities, and explicit respect for the other member of the treatment team are important ingredients. We are not aware of any studies formally comparing single- and two-provider forms of combined treatment.

Sequential combined treatment

Combined treatment also can be provided in sequence (Table 3.7). Results of one case control study suggested that it may be more efficient to provide IPT and pharmacotherapy in sequence rather than routinely start the therapies in combination. Specifically, 79% of the group treated with IPT followed, if indicated, by pharmacotherapy remitted, as compared with 66% of a historical comparison group that was treated with both IPT and imipramine from the outset of treatment. Conversely, the benefit of adding CT to antidepressant medications was demonstrated in three studies: two focusing on patients who obtained partial remission on antidepressants and one studying patients with highly recurrent depression who were being withdrawn from medication. In all three trials, CT reduced the risk of relapse and, in two of the studies, facilitated discontinuation of antidepressants.

The preventive effects of a modified form of group CBT emphasizing the use of mindfulness-based cognitive therapy strategies (MBCT) was compared to treatment as usual (TAU) for relapse prevention in unmedicated patients who had recovered from a recent episode of recurrent depression. Among those who

Table 3.7 Recommendations for sequential combined treatment. Sequential application of therapies (i.e. adding psychotherapy following partial response to pharmacotherapy) may be an effective strategy

Therapeutic choice	Recommendations	Evidence
First	Adding CT to treat residual depressive symptoms after acute treatment with pharmacotherapy improves remission rates and reduces relapse/recurrence rates	Level 2
	Adding pharmacotherapy for women with partial or no response after acute treatment with IPT improves remission rates	Level 3

had suffered from three or more lifetime episodes of depression, relapse risk was reduced from 66% in the TAU condition to 37% in the MBCT condition.

Conclusions

There is sufficient evidence to consider three forms of depression-focused psychotherapy (CT, BT and IPT) to be effective treatments for mild-to-moderately severe, nonbipolar depressive disorders. When available and pre-ferred by the patient, these therapies may be first choice interventions. Concurrent depression-focused psychotherapies also increase the effective-ness of pharmacotherapy for patients with severe, recurrent or chronic depression. Sequential application of treatments is a possible alternative. Although long-term enduring benefits have not been definitively estab-lished, some evidence does support preventive effects following termination of CT or with continuation of CT or IPT.

Bibliography

Bandura A, Adams NE, Beyer J. Cognitive processes mediating behavioral change. *J Pers Soc Psychol* 1977; **35**: 125–39.

Beach SR, Fincham FD, Katz J. Marital therapy in the treatment of depression: toward a third generation of therapy and research. *Clin Psychol Rev* 1998; **18**: 635–61.

Beck AT, Greenberg RL. *Coping with Depression*. New York (NY): Institute for Rational Living, 1974.

Beck AT, Rush AJ, Shaw BF, Emery G. *Cognitive Therapy of Depression*. New York: Guilford Press, 1979.

Bellack AS, Hersen M, Himmelhoch J. Social skills training compared with pharmaco-therapy and psychotherapy in the treatment of unipolar depression. *Am J Psychiatry* 1981; **138**: 1562–7.

Blackburn IM, Bishop S, Glen AI *et al*. The efficacy of cognitive therapy in depression: a treatment trial using cognitive therapy and pharmacotherapy, each alone and in combination. *Br J Psychiatry* 1981; **139**: 181–9.

Burns DD. *The Feeling Good Handbook*. New York: Plume, 1999.

Cuijpers P. Bibliotherapy in unipolar depression: a meta-analysis. *J Behav Ther Exp Psychiatry* 1997; **28**: 139–47.

DeRubeis RJ, Crits-Christoph P. Empirically supported individual and group psycho-logical treatments for adult mental disorders. *J Consult Clin Psychol* 1998; **66**: 37–52.

DeRubeis RJ, Gelfand LA, Tang TZ, Simons AD. Medications versus cognitive behavior therapy for severely depressed outpatients: mega-analysis of four randomized comparisons. *Am J Psychiatry* 1999; **156**: 1007–13.

Elkin I, Shea MT, Watkins JT *et al*. National Institute of Mental Health Treatment of Depression Collaborative Research Program. General effectiveness of treatments. *Arch Gen Psychiatry* 1989; **46**: 971–82.

Frank E, Grochocinski VJ, Spanier CA *et al*. Interpersonal psychotherapy and anti-depressant medication: evaluation of a sequential treatment strategy in women with recurrent major depression. *J Clin Psychiatry* 2000; **61**: 51–7.

Freud S. Mourning and melancholia. In: Strachey J (ed.) *The Standard Edition of the Complete Psychological Works of Sigmund Freud*, Vol. 20. London: Hogarth Press, 1957, pp 87–174.

Gloaguen V, Cottraux J, Cucherat M, Blackburn IM. A meta-analysis of the effects of cognitive therapy in depressed patients. *J Affect Disord* 1998; **49**: 59–72.

Greenberger D, Padesky CA. *Mind Over Mood*. New York: Guilford Press, 1995.

Hollon SD, DeRubeis RJ, Evans MD *et al*. Cognitive therapy and pharmacotherapy for depression. Singly and in combination. *Arch Gen Psychiatry* 1992; **49**: 774–81.

Keller MB, McCullough JP, Klein DN *et al*. A comparison of nefazodone, the cognitive behavioral-analysis system of psychotherapy, and their combination for the treatment of chronic depression. *N Engl J Med* 2000; **342**: 1462–70.

Klerman GL, Weissman MM, Rounsaville BJ, Chevron ES. *Interpersonal Psychotherapy of Depression*. New York: Basic Books, 1984.

Kovacs M, Rush AJ, Beck AT, Hollon SD. Depressed outpatients treated with cognitive therapy or pharmacotherapy. A one-year follow-up. *Arch Gen Psychiatry* 1981; **38**: 33–9.

Loizzo J. Meditation and psychotherapy. In: Muskin P (ed.) *Review of Psychiatry*, Vol. 19. Washington DC: American Psychiatric Association Press, 2000.

Markowitz JC, Svartberg M, Swartz HA. Is IPT time-limited psychodynamic psycho-therapy? *J Psychother Pract Res* 1998; **7**: 185–95.

McCullough JP. *Treatment of Chronic Depression*. New York: Guilford Press, 2000.

McRoberts C, Burlingame GM, Hoag MJ. Comparative efficacy of individual and group psychotherapy: a meta-analytic perspective. *Group Dynamics: Theory, Research, and Practice* 1998; **2**: 101–17.

Ravindran AV, Anisman H, Merali Z *et al*. Treatment of primary dysthymia with group cognitive therapy and pharmacotherapy: clinical symptoms and functional impairments. *Am J Psychiatry* 1999; **156**: 1608–17.

Reynolds CF III, Frank E, Perel JM *et al*. High relapse rate after discontinuation of adjunctive medication for elderly patients with recurrent major depression. *Am J Psychiatry* 1996; **153**: 1418–22.

Segal ZV, Kennedy SH, Cohen NL, the CANMAT Depression Work Group. Clinical guidelines for the treatment of depressive disorders. V. Combining psychotherapy and pharmacotherapy. *Can J Psychiatry* 2001; **46** (Suppl. 1): 59S–62S.

Segal ZV, Whitney DK, Lam RW, the CANMAT Depression Work Group. Clinical guidelines for the treatment of depressive disorders. III. Psychotherapy. *Can J Psychiatry* 2001; **46** (Suppl. 1): 29S–37S.

Simons AD, Murphy GE, Levine JL, Wetzel RD. Cognitive therapy and pharmacotherapy for depression. Sustained improvement over one year. *Arch Gen Psychiatry* 1986; **43**: 43–8.

Svartberg M, Stiles TC. Comparative effects of short-term psychodynamic psychotherapy: a meta-analysis. *J Consult Clin Psychol* 1991; **59**: 704–14.

Teasdale JD, Segal ZV, Williams JM *et al*. Prevention of relapse/recurrence in major depression by mindfulness-based cognitive therapy. *J Consult Clin Psychol* 2000; **68**: 615–23.

Thase ME. When are psychotherapy and pharmacotherapy combinations the treatment of choice for major depressive disorder? *Psychiatr Q* 1999; **70**: 333–46.

Thase ME, Simons AD, Cahalane J *et al*. Severity of depression and response to cognitive behavior therapy. *Am J Psychiatry* 1991; **148**: 784–9.

Thase ME, Greenhouse JB, Frank E *et al*. Treatment of major depression with psychotherapy or psychotherapy–pharmacotherapy combinations. *Arch Gen Psychiatry* 1997; **54**: 1009–15.

Weissman MM, Markowitz JC, Klerman GL. *A Comprehensive Guide to Interpersonal Psychotherapy*. New York: Basic Books, 2000.

Chapter 4

Evolution of antidepressant agents

In the beginning …

All currently available antidepressants fit into one of three pharmacological classes (Figure 4.1). In each class the first or prototypical drug was discovered empirically. For the first two classes, this was as a result of astute clinical observation of patients who were receiving the drugs for other disorders: tuberculosis (TB) in the case of the monoamine oxidase inhibitors (MAOIs) and schizophrenia in the case of the tricyclic antidepressants (TCAs). In the third class, the discovery was made on the basis of animal studies with agents that showed similar behavioural properties to established drugs, despite different pharmacological mechanisms.

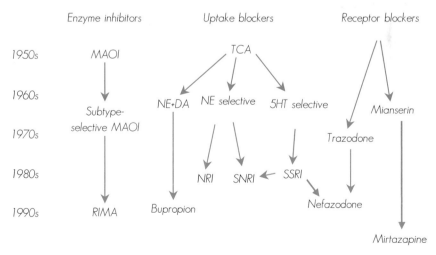

Figure 4.1 Evolution of antidepressants. (MAOI, monoamine oxidase inhibitor; RIMA, reversible inhibitor of monoamine oxidase A; NE, norepinephrine; 5HT, serotonin; TCA, tricyclic antidepressant; DA, dopamine; SSRI, selective serotonin re-uptake inhibitor; NRI, norepinephrine re-uptake inhibitor; SNRI, selective norepinephrine re-uptake inhibitor)

Since these empirical and serendipitous beginnings, each class of antidepressant drug therapy has undergone major growth and refinement. The biggest gains have been in the areas of increased tolerability and safety; in terms of efficacy the gains have been less apparent.

Enzyme inhibitors

The monoamine oxidase inhibitors (MAOIs)

This was the first class of antidepressants to be identified. In the late 1940s isoniazid and related compounds were used to treat TB patients, many of whom experienced a sense of elation even though they were experiencing little or no improvement in their physical health. This led to early clinical trials and the use of these drugs in depressed patients with considerable success.

At the same time it became known that the link between all these drugs was the property of inhibiting the enzyme MAO, hence the name MAOIs. This enzyme blockade prevents the degradation of amines especially serotonin (5HT) and norepinephrine (NE). By the 1960s it was recognized that there were two forms of MAO, type A and type B, both of which were irreversibly blocked by the MAOI antidepressants.

Because the type A enzyme is responsible for the metabolism of NE and 5HT this became the main target for antidepressant drug development. Selective but irreversible MAO-A antagonists such as pargyline were tested but they were disappointing as antidepressants, so were not licenced. Later the selective and irreversible MAO-B antagonist selegiline was synthesized and shown to be of use in Parkinson's disease, probably because dopamine is mostly metabolized by the B form of the enzyme.

Reversible MAOIs

The next step in the evolution of the MAOIs came with the development of the RIMA agents such as moclobemide and befloxatone. The acronym is derived from *r*eversible *i*nhibitor of *m*onoamine oxidase *A*. Conventional MAOIs destroy the MAO enzyme by binding to it irreversibly. As a consequence little enzyme is left to metabolize other amines, such as tyramine, found in many foods and medicines. High concentrations of tyramine are found in fermented meat, yeast preparations and mature dairy products. Tyramine is usually metabolized by MAO in the gut wall and liver so little enters the body. However, MAOIs stop this local breakdown, allowing tyramine to enter the central nervous system where it is taken up into amine neurons and displaces neurotransmitter monoamines from their storage vesicles. When large amounts of tyramine are ingested, a massive release of amines can occur with potentially disastrous consequences due to increased blood pressure and hyperthermia – the 'cheese reaction'.

By contrast, RIMAs do not permanently inactivate the MAO enzyme. They simply compete with amines at the active site of the enzyme. This means that, in the presence of rising tyramine levels, the RIMA agent will be displaced, freeing the enzyme to break down potentially harmful tyramine. Moreover, as RIMAs only block the A form of the enzyme and tyramine is a substrate for both A and B enzyme, there is plenty of spare MAO to complete the metabolism.

The RIMAs are fairly safe drugs although a mild cheese reaction can be observed, particularly at higher than recommended doses (in the case of moclobemide, this means a daily dose of 900 mg or more). There are also risks of interactions with sympathomimetic drugs such as cold cures, and the serotonin syndrome has been observed when moclobemide is combined with a selective serotonin reuptake inhibitor (SSRI).

Amine uptake blocking agents

The tricyclic antidepressants (TCAs)

Imipramine is a derivative of the first antipsychotic chlorpromazine. In the late 1950s it was tested in schizophrenia: it had little effect on the psychotic symptoms but was observed to elevate mood. Soon imipramine and its close relative amitriptyline were tested in depressed patients and found to have good efficacy.

In 1964 Iversen and colleagues showed that imipramine prevented the uptake of tritiated NE into brain tissue. This heralded the beginning of the 'neurotransmitter/transporter' era in pharmacology with the subsequent discovery of different families of transporters that regulate neurotransmitter concentrations in the synaptic cleft. These transporters are targets for a variety of psychotropic dugs. It also contributed to the emerging NE theory of depression and antidepressant drug action, as several TCAs such as nortriptyline and protriptyline were NE selective uptake blockers. In recent years, several NE reuptake inhibitors (NRIs) of nontricyclic structure have been developed. These include maprotiline and reboxetine as well as the NE/dopamine uptake blockers bupropion and nomifensine. Nomifensine was withdrawn worldwide in the mid-1990s due to an unacceptably high incidence of hematological adverse effects, but these other agents will be discussed in later chapters (see Chapters 5 and 6).

The selective serotonin reuptake inhibitors (SSRIs)

The next advance occurred when Carlsson and Ross observed that the TCAs also blocked the uptake of 5HT into synaptosomes. This provided support for the 5HT theory of depression and suggested that selective 5HT uptake blockers might also be antidepressant. The effectiveness of clomipramine, a relatively 5HT-selective TCA, supported this view but the real breakthrough came with the synthesis and testing of the first SSRI, zimelidine. Even though it had a totally different profile of side-effects compared with the TCAs and was safe in overdose, zimelidine's useful life was cut short by reports of rare but severe hepatitis and Guillain–Barré syndrome. The company that developed it thought that these adverse effects were a consequence of blocking 5HT reuptake and discontinued their SSRI development program. However, other companies took a different view and were later proved correct with the development of a series of SSRIs that have proved to be exceptionally safe and effective antidepressant and anxiolytic agents.

Although efficacy and side-effects across drugs in the SSRI class are generally similar, there are some pharmacological distinctions. Citalopram selectively blocks the 5HT transporter (SERT), paroxetine blocks SERT and to a lesser extent the NE transporter, while sertraline mainly blocks SERT and has a minor blocking effect on the DA transporter.

Dual-action antidepressants

In recent years the potential advantages of dual 5HT and NE reuptake blockade compared with either alone have been reported. Firstly, the Danish University Antidepressant Group conducted three studies that compared the TCA clomipramine at high doses with paroxetine, citalopram and moclobemide in severely depressed hospitalized patients. In each study clomipramine showed superior efficacy, which they attributed to the NE uptake blocking properties of a metabolite of clomipramine as well as the 5HT-blocking properties of the parent compound. Secondly, Nelson *et al.* (1991) showed that an SSRI (fluoxetine) combined with a NRI (desipramine) produced a more rapid outcome than fluoxetine alone.

These findings have supported the development of the dual-action non-TCA uptake blockers venlafaxine and duloxetine. In a series of meta-analyses, venlafaxine has been shown to have superior response and remission rates compared with the SSRIs in depressed patients. It should be noted, however, that remission rates for SSRIs in these comparison studies are generally lower than those reported in other SSRI trials. Hence the issue remains controversial and requires adequately powered trials to compare remission rates between SSRI and SNRI agents. Interestingly among the SSRI class, paroxetine has been suggested to have dual 5HT and NE effects '*in vitro*' (a finding that distinguishes it from other SSRIs, though the main metabolite of fluoxetine, norfluoxetine, is also somewhat of an NE uptake blocker). In one study, paroxetine was shown to have comparable efficacy to TCAs in hospitalized patients. There is also evidence that mirtazapine, which promotes 5HT and NE transmission, has superior efficacy to SSRIs in severely depressed patients.

Milnacipran is available in France and Japan. It displays greater NE than 5HT-blocking effects – the opposite of venlafaxine. This dual-uptake blocking drug has been shown to be effective in a number of clinical trials in depression. Early data suggest it may show increased efficacy compared with SSRIs such as fluoxetine.

Duloxetine is the newest member of this class. It is a more potent dual reuptake inhibitor than venlafaxine. At a standard dose of 60 mg daily, blockade of both 5HT and NE transporters has been reported. In contrast, venlafaxine requires a dose increase from 75 to 150 mg for comparable NE blockade to occur. Preliminary reports confirm higher rates of remission when duloxetine was compared with fluoxetine. Interestingly, both duloxetine and venlafaxine appear to have beneficial effects on physical pain, a property they share with amitriptyline but not SSRIs. Duloxetine appears to have a role in treating neuropathic pain. These findings support claims for an SNRI class effect including higher remission rates and 'broad spectrum' efficacy.

There are interesting theoretical reasons why an antidepressant that acts on more than one transmitter system might have superior efficacy. Although increasing the actions of either 5HT or NE is an effective way to treat depression, there is some evidence that these two transmitter systems have rather different effects on the various physical and emotional functions that are disrupted in depression (Figure 4.2).

Although there is considerable overlap between transmitters and symptoms, some symptoms are more relevant to either 5HT or NE. The implication of this differentiation of transmitter functions is that certain

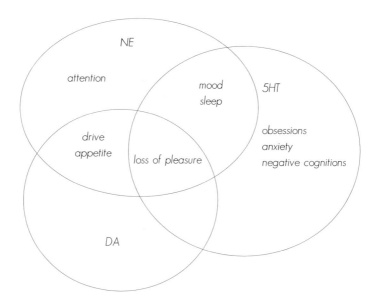

Figure 4.2 Neurotransmitters and depressive symptoms.

antidepressants might preferentially treat some depressive symptoms and not others. So an NE-enhancing antidepressant might be preferred in individuals who are lacking in energy, drive or attention, whereas a more 5HT-targeting drug would be preferred in patients with prominent obsessional or anxiety symptoms. Dual-action agents or triple-action would be effective across more than one symptom cluster.

Receptor acting drugs

These are the third class of antidepressants, and again they were discovered before a theory of action was developed. The first two drugs in this class, (mianserin and trazodone) were both found to have antidepressant activity in animal and other preclinical models of antidepressant action. On this basis they were taken into human trials where they proved effective. Subsequent animal studies helped unravel their mode of action although it should be said that this issue is still debated.

The first theory to explain the therapeutic actions of mianserin was that of α_2-adrenoceptor antagonism. This fitted with emerging ideas about antidepressant mechanisms for other treatments, such as TCAs and electroconvulsive therapy (ECT). A decrease in α_2-adrenoceptor function would remove autoinhibition of NE neurons so increasing NE concentration in the synaptic cleft. Based on this theory, mirtazapine and other α_2-adrenoceptor antagonists (e.g. fluparoxan and idazoxan) were evaluated in clinical trials. Only mirtazapine proved to be both effective and well tolerated, possibly because it is also a $5HT_2$ and $5HT_3$ receptor antagonist.

Mianserin (available in many European countries but not in the USA or Canada) and trazodone also interact with 5HT receptors. Mianserin antagonizes $5HT_{1A}$ and $5HT_{2C}$ receptors whereas trazodone acts through its own $5HT_2$-blocking effects and through its metabolite mCPP, which has $5HT_1$ and $5HT_{2C}$ agonist properties. Both are prototypes for antidepressants in this class. Mirtazapine is a refinement of mianserin with $5HT_2$ and $5HT_3$ receptor-blocking activity, which likely explains the virtual absence of 5HT-mediated side-effects such as headache, sexual dysfunction, insomnia and nausea. Mirtazapine also has less α_1-adrenoceptor blocking affinity than mianserin but is a potent histamine H_1 receptor blocker, so both agents promote sleep and can cause daytime sedation especially early in treatment. Nefazodone is a follow-up compound of trazodone that is a weak 5HT uptake blocker and a potent $5HT_2$ receptor antagonist. Its side-effect profile is distinct from the SSRIs based on less sexual dysfunction and sleep disturbance. However, its use has recently been restricted to named patients in some countries due to reported cases of hepatotoxicity.

Delayed onset of antidepressant action

One of the goals of antidepressant discovery has been the development of compounds with a faster onset of action. The prevailing view of the typical three to four week therapeutic delay with most antidepressants is that it takes this long to disable compensatory receptor-based mechanisms that initially offset the uptake blockade or amine oxidase inhibition. To some extent the receptor-blocking drugs should be free of this problem, although clinical data have been equivocal. For example, mirtazapine does seem to produce significantly greater improvements in mood and anxiety symptoms as well as sleep compared with SSRIs during the first two weeks of treatment, although these differences are not sustained after six to eight weeks of treatment.

A targeted approach to this issue came from animal studies in which blockade of the presynaptic $5HT_{1A}$ autoreceptor by antagonists such as pindolol produced a rapid rise in 5HT in cortex. However, a clinical trial program to test combined SSRI/pindolol therapy (with both fluoxetine and paroxetine) failed to produce support for the approach. This may have been because pindolol also blocks the postsynaptic $5HT_{1A}$ receptor, which likely needs to be stimulated to mediate the antidepressant cascade (Figures 4.3 and 4.4).

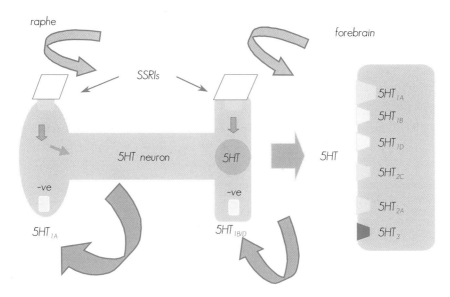

Figure 4.3 Effect of uptake blockade at the serotonergic synapse.

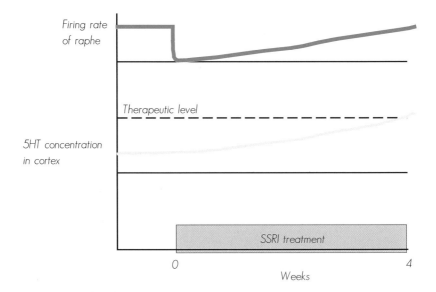

Figure 4.4 Time lag of SSRIs.

Conclusions

Many antidepressants have been discovered through serendipity. However, intense research efforts over the past 50 years have led to a better understanding of their pharmacology and to a growing insight into the way in which this pharmacology leads to adaptive brain changes that alleviate depression. All three classes of antidepressants have been subject to significant refinements in drug action, resulting in improved adverse effect and safety profile. Current evidence supports the recruitment of more than one neurotransmitter system to address the range of symptoms associated with MDD. An understanding of the pharmacology of antidepressants can improve their use both as single agents and when combined with other antidepressants in cases of treatment resistance, partial response and unwelcome adverse effects.

Bibliography

Beasley CM Jr, Nilsson ME, Koke SC, Gonzales JS. Efficacy, adverse events, and treatment discontinuations in fluoxetine clinical studies of major depression: a meta-analysis of the 20-mg/day dose. *J Clin Psychiatry* 2000; **61**: 722–8.

Carlsson A, Corrodi H, Fuxe K, Hokfelt T. Effect of antidepressant drugs on the depletion of intraneuronal brain 5-hydroxytryptamine stores caused by 4-alpha-ethyl-metatyramine. *Eur J Pharmacology* 1969; **5**: 357–66.

Clerc G. Antidepressant efficacy and tolerability of milnacipran, a dual serotonin and noradrenaline reuptake inhibitor: a comparison with fluvoxamine. *Int Clin Psychopharmacol* 2001; **16**(3): 145–51.

Healy D. *The Antidepressant Era*. Cambridge, Mass: Harvard University Press, 1997.

Iversen LL. *The Uptake and Storage of Noradrenaline in Sympathetic Nerves*. London: Cambridge University Press, 1967.

Nelson JC, Mazure CM, Bowers MB Jr, Jatlow PI. A preliminary, open study of the combination of fluoxetine and desipramine for rapid treatment of major depression. *Arch Gen Psychiatry* 1991; **48**: 303–7.

Nutt D. Mirtazapine: pharmacology in relation to adverse effects. *Acta Psychiatr Scand* 1997; **96** (Suppl. 391): 31–7.

Nutt DJ, Glue P. Clinical pharmacology of anxiolytics and antidepressants: a psychopharmacological perspective. In: File S (ed.) *Psychopharmacology of Anxiolytics and Antidepressants*. New York: Pergamon Press, 1991, pp 1–28.

Ross SB, Renyi AL. Inhibition of the uptake of tritiated 5-hydroxytryptamine in brain tissue. *Eur J Pharmacology* 1969; **7**: 270–7.

Smith D, Dempster C, Glanville J *et al.* Efficacy and tolerability of venlafaxine compared with selective serotonin reuptake inhibitors and other antidepressants: a meta-analysis. *Br J Psychiatry* 2002; **180**: 396–404.

Stahl SM, Entsuah R, Rudolph RL. Comparative efficacy between venlafaxine and SSRIs: a pooled analysis of patients with depression. *Biol Psychiatry* 2002; **52**: 1166–74.

Thase ME. Treatment of severe depression. *J Clin Psychiatry* 2000; **61** (Suppl. 1): 17–25.

Thase ME, Entsuah AR, Rudolph RL. Remission rates during treatment with venlafaxine or selective serotonin reuptake inhibitors. *Br J Psychiatry* 2001; **178**: 234–41.

Chapter 5

Therapeutic choices of antidepressants across depressive disorders

Criteria for choosing an antidepressant

Cornerstones in the decision-making process to choose an antidepressant are efficacy (inferred from randomized placebo-controlled trials or RCTs), tolerability (side-effect profiles) and safety (including overdose and drug combinations data). In developing these therapeutic choices for the treatment of depression we have superimposed expert opinion on an evidence-based review of these three dimensions (Tables 5.1 and 5.2).

Major depressive disorder

Selective serotonin reuptake inhibitors (SSRIs) and the dual-action agents have superior side-effect profiles and in most cases at least comparable efficacy to TCAs and MAOIs. This has resulted in their adoption as first-choice antidepressants for the treatment of major depressive disorder (MDD). Recent evidence has been presented to support higher rates of remission

Table 5.1 Criteria for levels of evidence

Level of evidence	Criteria
1	Meta-analysis or replicated RCT that includes a placebo condition
2	At least one RCT with placebo or active comparison condition
3	Uncontrolled trial with ten or more subjects
4	Anecdotal case reports

Table 5.2 Criteria for therapeutic choices

Therapeutic choice	Criteria
First	Level 1 or Level 2 evidence + clinical support
Second	Level 1, Level 2 or Level 3 evidence + clinical support
Third	Level 1, Level 2, Level 3 or Level 4 evidence + clinical support
Not recommended	Level 1 or Level 2 evidence for lack of efficacy, or insufficient information to evaluate efficacy

Table 5.3 Recommendations for treatment of MDD

Therapeutic choice	Recommendations	Evidence
First	SSRIs and dual-action agents (SNRI and others)	Level 1
	Venlafaxine and duloxetine have been reported to produce higher remission rates than SSRIs	Level 1
Second	Among TCAs amitriptyline and clomipramine have greater efficacy than SSRIs in hospitalized depressed patients (safety and tolerability issues need to be considered)	Level 2
Third	Other TCAs and MAOIs (lower recommendation because of safety and tolerability issues)	Level 2

for dual-action agents compared with SSRIs (Table 5.3). See Chapter 2 for definitions of response and remission.

Treatment options for subtypes of MDD

MDD exists in many clinical forms, which may reflect different biological and environmental disturbances. Clinicians recognize distinct subtypes of MDD, many of which are described in DSM-IV-R but not as distinctly in ICD-10 (see Chapter 1). Although evidence bases are limited in some cases, the following guidelines are offered for the pharmacological treatment of subtypes of MDD. As noted in the discussion of psychotherapies in MDD (Chapter 3), the absence of evidence for a particular antidepressant treatment should not be equated with evidence for lack of efficacy.

MDD with atypical features

The evidence to support one antidepressant or class of antidepressants over another is limited, mainly because there have been very few studies that focused exclusively on 'atypical depression'. Fluoxetine and imipramine were equally effective although fluoxetine was better tolerated in one trial. Sertraline and moclobemide were also effective for atypical depression, with some quality of life advantages for sertraline, while phenelzine was superior to imipramine (Table 5.4).

MDD with melancholic features

Although there is considerable overlap between 'melancholic depression', 'severe depression' (e.g. a score of 24 or more on the Hamilton Rating Scale for Depression) and depression requiring inpatient treatment these terms are not synonymous and treatment recommendations may not apply equally across groups.

There are conflicting claims about treatment superiority in melancholic patients. Clomipramine was associated with higher remission rates than sertraline, paroxetine and moclobemide in individual trials and a meta-analysis concluded that TCAs were superior to SSRIs but produced worse side-effects. Venlafaxine also produced higher remission rates compared with fluoxetine while nortriptyline was more effective than fluoxetine in an elderly melancholic population. However in separate meta-analyses paroxetine, moclobemide and venlafaxine were found to be comparable to TCAs (Table 5.5).

Table 5.4 Recommendations for treatment of MDD with atypical features

Therapeutic choice	Recommendations	Evidence
First	Fluoxetine; sertraline (and probably other SSRIs); moclobemide	Level 2
Second	Phenelzine (choice reduced due to poor tolerability)	Level 2
Third	Imipramine	Level 2

Table 5.5 Recommendations for treatment of MDD with melancholic features

Therapeutic choice	Recommendations	Evidence
First	Paroxetine; venlafaxine	Level 1
Second	TCAs, especially clomipramine	Level 1
Third	Citalopram; fluoxetine; moclobemide	Level 2

MDD with psychotic features: delusional depression

There are too few adequately powered trials to provide definitive recommendations. Most of the studies compare mixed psychotic and nonpsychotic depressed patients who received treatment under uncontrolled conditions. The combination of amitriptyline and perphenazine was significantly better than either alone. In a meta-analysis, electroconvulsive therapy (ECT) was superior to the TCA alone but was not significantly better than the combination of TCA and antipsychotic therapy. On the other hand, bilateral ECT was more effective than unilateral ECT. There was also a trend for combination TCA and antipsychotic treatment to be more effective than either medication alone. Results of this meta-analysis are limited by the inclusion of open-label trials and the use of older, typical antipsychotic medications. Although SSRI monotherapy (sertraline and paroxetine) has been reported to be effective in delusional depression, the use of SSRI monotherapy does not have widespread clinical acceptance.

The indications for novel antipsychotics (particularly olanzapine, risperidone and quetiapine) extend beyond psychotic disorders and into mood disorders. Emerging studies support their role in both psychotic depression and treatment-resistant depression (Table 5.6; see also Chapter 9, Table 9.2).

MDD with seasonal pattern: winter depression

Clinical guidelines for winter depression support light therapy as the first-choice therapy. Among the antidepressants that have been evaluated, fluoxetine and moclobemide are effective, while bupropion, citalopram and tranylcypromine were beneficial in open trials (Table 5.7). Results of studies

Table 5.6 Recommendations for treatment of MDD with psychotic features

Therapeutic choice	Recommendations	Evidence
First	Electroconvulsive therapy (ECT)	Level 1
	Antipsychotic + antidepressant (olanzapine or risperidone with SSRI or SNRI)	Level 2
Second	Typical antipsychotic + amitriptyline	Level 2
Not recommended	Monotherapy with SSRIs	Level 2 but limited clinical support

Table 5.7 Recommendations for treatment of MDD with seasonal pattern

Therapeutic choice	Recommendations	Evidence
First	Bright light therapy	Level 1
Second	Fluoxetine; moclobemide	Level 2
Third	Bupropion; citalopram; tranylcypromine	Level 3

comparing light therapy, antidepressants and the combination are not yet available.

'Anxious depression'

Although 'anxious depression' is not specified as a subtype of MDD within DSM-IV-TR, the majority (60–90%) of individuals with a primary diagnosis of depression also experience symptoms of anxiety and 30–50% of MDD patients suffer from at least one comorbid anxiety disorder. Individuals who suffer from 'anxious depression' have greater severity of depressive symptomatology, greater functional and psychosocial impairment, higher suicide risk and poorer prognosis following treatment, compared with depressed individuals with low levels of anxiety. Most SSRIs and venlafaxine have proven efficacy in the treatment of anxiety disorders, which supports their use in anxious depression.

In three meta-analyses, moclobemide, mirtazapine and venlafaxine were as effective as active comparators (imipramine, amitriptyline and trazodone) and superior to placebo. Paroxetine and sertraline were as effective as clomipramine, while fluvoxamine and lorazepam were comparable in efficacy. Other studies also support the efficacy of paroxetine in reducing symptoms of anxiety associated with depression. Clonazepam augmentation of fluoxetine was superior to fluoxetine alone in the first three weeks of a double-blind trial, although dependency concerns restrict recommendations for concurrent benzodiazepine prescription (Table 5.8).

Treatment options for chronic depression/dysthymic disorder

Dysthymic disorder and double depression (a major depressive episode superimposed on dysthymia) are often indistinguishable. For some patients,

Table 5.8 Recommendations for treatment of 'anxious depression'

Therapeutic choice	Recommendations	Evidence
First	Mirtazapine; moclobemide; paroxetine; sertraline; venlafaxine	Level 1
Second	Amitriptyline; fluvoxamine; imipramine; trazodone	Level 1
Not recommended	Lorazepam or other benzodiazepines are not recommended as monotherapy due to lack of efficacy and concerns about dependency, but may be used as short-term adjunctive therapies	Level 2

the duration of symptoms may be as long as 30 years prior to treatment. Despite the limited number of trials, there is general agreement that pharmacological treatments are more effective than placebo in the acute treatment of patients with dysthymia. In a meta-analysis, fluoxetine, sertraline, MAOIs including moclobemide and TCAs all had equivalent efficacy, although TCAs were associated with more side-effects and higher dropout rates. There were no significant differences in rates of response between patients with pure dysthymia and those with double depression. For this reason, the term 'chronic depression' is often used.

Sertraline is the most investigated SSRI for chronic depression and had advantages over imipramine. In patients over the age of 60, who were treated in primary care settings, paroxetine was superior to placebo. Overall, data from clinical trials suggest no differences in dose range, frequency of adverse effects or placebo response in the treatment of chronic depression/dysthymic disorder compared to MDD. Venlafaxine and mirtazapine were also effective in open trials (Table 5.9). Combined pharmacotherapy with nefazodone and

Table 5.9 Recommendations for treatment of chronic depression/dysthymic disorder

Therapeutic choice	Recommendations	Evidence
First	Fluoxetine; fluvoxamine; moclobemide; nefazodone; paroxetine; sertraline	Level 2
Second	Desipramine; imipramine	Level 2
Third	Mirtazapine; venlafaxine	Level 3

a modified form of CBT – Cognitive Behavioural Analysis System of Psychotherapy (CBASP) – produced superior results compared to either treatment alone (see Chapter 3).

Other depressive disorders

Minor depressive disorder (mDD)

Patients who meet criteria for mDD have fewer symptoms than MDD patients but may be equally impaired. Most patients remain in primary care settings and are rarely seen by psychiatrists. There is most evidence to support the use of paroxetine in mDD. Paroxetine and problem-solving treatment were both superior to placebo in a primary care trial in patients over 60 years of age, and paroxetine was superior to maprotiline in a middle life population. Fluvoxamine was associated with a significant decrease in depressive symptomatology and an improvement in psychosocial functioning in an open-label trial (Table 5.10).

Recurrent brief depression

In recurrent brief depression, the number and severity of symptoms are comparable to MDD but the duration is shorter: at least two days but less than two weeks. Despite favourable case reports including case series on the effectiveness of fluoxetine, mirtazapine, reboxetine and tranylcypromine, neither fluoxetine nor paroxetine was superior to placebo under controlled conditions. Timing of rating scale assessments in these trials may account for the negative results (Table 5.11).

Conclusions

In most cases, patients with different forms of depression can be treated effectively with a variety of different antidepressants. The main influences

Table 5.10 Recommendations for treatment of mDD

Therapeutic choice	Recommendations	Evidence
First	Paroxetine (based on individuals aged 60 years and older)	Level 2
Second	Fluvoxamine	Level 3
	Maprotiline	Level 2

Table 5.11 Recommendations for antidepressant treatment of recurrent brief depression

Therapeutic choice	Recommendation	Evidence
Not recommended	No available support for antidepressant treatment	Level 2

on choice of antidepressant are drug tolerability and the evidence base in the specific syndrome under treatment. It seems likely that differences between drugs used in the different syndromes emerge from variations in their pharmacology but this is not yet proved.

Bibliography

Ackermann RT, Williams JW Jr. Rational treatment choices for non-major depressions in primary care: an evidence-based review. *J Gen Intern Med* 2002; **17**: 293–301.

American Psychiatric Association. *Diagnostic and Statistical Manual of Mental Disorders*, 4th edn, Text Revision (DSM-IV-TR). Washington DC: American Psychiatric Press, 2000.

Bauer M, Whybrow PC, Angst J *et al*. World Federation of Societies of Biological Psychiatry (WFSBP) Guidelines for Biological Treatment of Unipolar Depressive Disorders. Part 1. Acute and continuation treatment of major depressive disorder. *World J Biol Psychiatry* 2002; **3**: 5–43.

Bauer M, Whybrow PC, Angst J *et al*. World Federation of Societies of Biological Psychiatry (WFSBP) Guidelines for Biological Treatment of Unipolar Depressive Disorders. Part 2. Maintenance treatment of major depressive disorder and treatment of chronic depressive disorders and subthreshold depressions. *World J Biol Psychiatry* 2002; **3**: 69–86.

Benkert O, Muller M, Szegedi A. An overview of the clinical efficacy of mirtazapine. *Hum Psychopharmacol* 2002; **17** (Suppl. 1): S23–S26.

Clerc GE, Ruimy P, Verdeau-Palles J. A double-blind comparison of venlafaxine and fluoxetine in patients hospitalized for major depression and melancholia. The Venlafaxine French Inpatient Study Group. *Int Clin Psychopharmacol* 1994; **9**: 139–43.

De Lima MS, Hotopf M. Benefits and risks of pharmacotherapy for dysthymia: a systematic appraisal of the evidence. *Drug Saf* 2003; **26**: 55–64.

De Lima MS, Hotopf M, Wessely S. The efficacy of drug treatments for dysthymia: a systematic review and meta-analysis. *Psychol Med* 1999; **29**: 1273–89.

Dewan MJ, Anand VS. Evaluating the tolerability of the newer antidepressants. *J Nerv Ment Dis* 1999; **187**: 96–101.

Keller MB, McCullough JP, Klein DN *et al.* A comparison of nefazodone, the cognitive behavioral-analysis system of psychotherapy, and their combination for the treatment of chronic depression. *N Engl J Med* 2000; **342**: 1462–70.

Kennedy SH, Eisfeld BS, Meyer JH, Bagby RM. Antidepressants in clinical practice: limitations of assessment methods and drug response. *Hum Psychopharmacol* 2001; **16**: 105–14.

Kennedy SH, Lam RW, Cohen NL, Ravindran AV, the CANMAT Depression Work Group. Clinical guidelines for the treatment of depressive disorders. IV. Medications and other biological treatments. *Can J Psychiatry* 2001; **46** (Suppl. 1): 38S–58S.

Lam RW, Levitt AJ. *Canadian Consensus Guidelines for the Treatment of Seasonal Affective Disorder.* Vancouver, BC: Clinical & Academic Publishing, 1999.

McGrath PJ, Stewart JW, Janal MN *et al.* A placebo-controlled study of fluoxetine versus imipramine in the acute treatment of atypical depression. *Am J Psychiatry* 2000; **157**: 344–50.

Montgomery DB, Roberts A, Green M *et al.* Lack of efficacy of fluoxetine in recurrent brief depression and suicidal attempts. *Eur Arch Psychiatry Clin Neurosci* 1994; **244**: 211–15.

Ninan PT, Berger J. Symptomatic and syndromal anxiety and depression. *Depress Anxiety* 2001; **14**: 79–85.

Oxman TE, Sengupta A. Treatment of minor depression. *Am J Geriatr Psychiatry* 2002; **10**: 256–64.

Pezawas L, Angst J, Gamma A *et al.* Recurrent brief depression – past and future. *Prog Neuropsychopharmacol Biol Psychiatry* 2003; **27**: 75–83.

Quitkin FM, McGrath PJ, Stewart JW *et al.* Atypical depression, panic attacks, and response to imipramine and phenelzine. A replication. *Arch Gen Psychiatry* 1990; **47**: 935–41.

Rapaport MH, Judd LL. Minor depressive disorder and subsyndromal depressive symptoms: functional impairment and response to treatment. *J Affect Disord* 1998; **48**: 227–32.

Ravindran AV, Guelfi JD, Lane RM, Cassano GB. Treatment of dysthymia with sertraline: a double-blind, placebo-controlled trial in dysthymic patients without major depression. *J Clin Psychiatry* 2000; **61**: 821–7.

Roose SP, Glassman AH, Attia E, Woodring S. Comparative efficacy of selective serotonin reuptake inhibitors and tricyclics in the treatment of melancholia. *Am J Psychiatry* 1994; **151**: 1735–9.

Rothschild AJ. Challenges in the treatment of depression with psychotic features. *Biol Psychiatry* 2003; **53**: 680–90.

Smith D, Dempster C, Glanville J *et al.* Efficacy and tolerability of venlafaxine compared with selective serotonin reuptake inhibitors and other antidepressants: a meta-analysis. *Br J Psychiatry* 2002; **180**: 396–404.

Sogaard J, Lane R, Latimer P *et al*. A 12-week study comparing moclobemide and sertraline in the treatment of outpatients with atypical depression. *J Psychopharmacol* 1999; **13**: 406–14.

Stahl SM, Entsuah R, Rudolph RL. Comparative efficacy between venlafaxine and SSRIs: a pooled analysis of patients with depression. *Biol Psychiatry* 2002; **52**: 1166–74.

Stamenkovic M, Blasbichier T, Riederer F *et al*. Fluoxetine treatment in patients with recurrent brief depression. *Int Clin Psychopharmacol* 2001; **16**: 221–6.

Szegedi A, Wetzel H, Angersbach D *et al*. Response to treatment in minor and major depression: results of a double-blind comparative study with paroxetine and maprotiline. *J Affect Disord* 1997; **45**: 167–78.

Thase ME, Fava M, Halbreich U *et al*. A placebo-controled, randomized clinical trial comparing sertraline and imipramine for the treatment of dysthymia. *Arch Gen Psychiatry* 1996; **53**: 777–84.

Thase ME, Entsuah AR, Rudolph RL. Remission rates during treatment with venlafaxine or selective serotonin reuptake inhibitors. *Br J Psychiatry* 2001; **178**: 234–41.

Thase ME, Nierenberg AA, Keller MB, Panagides J, the Relapse Prevention Study Group. Efficacy of mirtazapine for the prevention of depressive relapse: a placebo-controlled double-blind trial of recently remitted high-risk patients. *J Clin Psychiatry* 2001; **62**: 782–8.

Tignol J, Stoker MJ, Dunbar GC. Paroxetine in the treatment of melancholia and severe depression. *Int Clin Psychopharmacol* 1992; **7**: 91–4.

World Health Organization. *International Statistical Classification of Diseases and Related Health Problems*, Tenth Revision (ICD–10). Geneva: World Health Organization, 1992.

Zanardi R, Franchini L, Gasperini M *et al*. Double-blind controled trial of sertraline versus paroxetine in the treatment of delusional depression. *Am J Psychiatry* 1996; **153**: 1631–3.

Chapter 6

Practical issues in selecting antidepressants

Introduction

Clinicians should be aware of the different antidepressant classes and develop expertise in using one or two drugs from each class. Compliance is an important but frequently neglected aspect of antidepressant treatment and has a significant influence on treatment outcome. Variables other than side-effects can account for low rates of compliance. Stigma and a limited understanding of how antidepressants work are modifiable risk factors for noncompliance (see Chapter 2).

This chapter will deal with dosing, side-effects, drug interactions, overdose toxicity, prevention of recurrence and discontinuation issues. Some drugs are available in most countries although others, such as bupropion, milnacipran, reboxetine and tianeptine, have limited availability. Comparisons of side-effects across drugs and drug classes are limited by the absence of direct 'head-to-head' trials. In the absence of direct comparisons, we have selected those side-effects that occurred significantly more frequently ($\geq 10\%$ and $\geq 30\%$) compared with placebo.

The monoamine oxidase inhibitors (MAOIs)

The MAOIs continue to offer an important alternative therapeutic choice, particularly for treatment-resistant depression. In general it is important to initiate treatment at a low dose with gradual dose increments (Table 6.1).

The two main limitations of MAOIs are the high side-effect burden and concerns about food and drug interactions (Table 6.2). Dizziness and orthostatic hypotension are common to all MAOIs and are often dose related.

Table 6.1 Dosing of MAOIs

Drug	Dosage adjustment (mg)		
	Starting[1]	Usual	High[2]
Reversible			
Moclobemide	200-300	450-600	900
Irreversible			
Isocarboxazid	10-20	30-40	60
Phenelzine	15-30	45-75	90-120
Tranylcypromine	10-20	30-60	70-90

1. Lower starting dose indicated with previous sensitivity to side-effects or with polypharmacy; often applies to elderly patients.
2. Higher doses often exceed recommended upper limits in formularies; these doses should be used with caution.

Table 6.2 Frequently reported side-effects across MAOIs

Antidepressant	Incidence of side-effects		
	≥30%	≥10%	
Moclobemide	None	Insomnia	Blurred vision
		Excitement; hypomania	Orthostatic
		Headache	hypotension/dizziness
		Dry mouth	GI distress
Isocarboxazid	None	Headache	Orthostatic
		Dry mouth	hypotension/dizziness
		Tremor	GI distress
Phenelzine	Dry mouth	Drowsiness; sedation	Tremor
	Sexual	Insomnia	Orthostatic
	disturbances	Excitement; hypomania,	hypotension/dizziness
		Blurred vision	Tachycardia; palpitations
		Constipation	GI distress
		Extra-pyramidal side-effects	Weight gain (over 6 kg)
Tranylcypromine	None	Drowsiness; sedation	Orthostatic
		Insomnia	hypotension/dizziness
		Excitement; hypomania	Tachycardia; palpitations
		Dry mouth	

GI, gastrointestinal.

Insomnia and sexual dysfunction are also frequently encountered adverse events. However, the collection of data on side-effects for older antidepressants was less rigorous than would be required today, so accurate prevalences are difficult to establish. In clinical practice, side-effects can sometimes be minimized by altering the timing of dosing. For example, in cases where MAOIs taken in the morning disrupt sleep, switching to night-time dosing may reduce insomnia.

The tricyclic antidepressants (TCAs)

TCAs continue to be prescribed worldwide (Table 6.3). Amitriptyline, clomipramine and imipramine are the main mixed-uptake blocking agents (see Chapter 4). Although clomipramine is frequently used to treat hospitalized depressed patients in Europe, in the USA it is only indicated for the treatment of obsessive compulsive disorder. Amitriptyline continues to be used extensively for the management of chronic pain, although recent reports that dual-action antidepressants (duloxetine and venlafaxine) are effective in the treatment of pain, may decrease its usage. Desipramine and nortriptyline are TCAs that preferentially block norepinephrine (NE) reuptake. They respectively display linear and curvilinear dose–response

Table 6.3 Dosing of TCAs[1]

Drug	Dosage adjustment (mg)		
	Starting[2]	Usual	High[3]
Tertiary amines			
Amitriptyline	25-50	75-200	250-300
Clomipramine	50-75	100-250	300-450
Imipramine	50-75	100-250	300-450
Secondary amines			
Desipramine	25-50	75-150	200-300
Nortriptyline	25-50	75-150	200

1. These are five examples of TCAs; other available TCAs are doxepin, maprotiline, protriptyline and trimipramine.
2. Lower starting dose indicated with previous sensitivity to side-effects or with polypharmacy; often applies to elderly patients.
3. Higher doses often exceed recommended upper limits in formularies; these doses should be used with caution.

pharmacokinetics. Therefore plasma levels should be monitored to ensure optimal dosing.

A major concern with TCAs relates to their multiple receptor targets beyond NE or 5HT transporters, especially the cholinergic muscarinic, α_1-adrenergic and histamine H_1 receptors. Antagonism of these receptors can produce a disparate array of side-effects: anticholinergic and cardiovascular effects are the most prevalent, especially in elderly patients. Side-effects for the most frequently prescribed TCAs are reviewed in Table 6.4.

Table 6.4 Frequently reported side-effects across TCAs

Antidepressant	Incidence of side-effects		
	≥ 30%	≥ 10%	
Amitriptyline	Drowsiness; sedation	Disorientation/confusion	Tremor
	Dry mouth	Asthenia; fatigue	Orthostatic
	Weight gain	Blurred vision	hypotension/dizziness
	(over 6 kg)	Constipation	Tachycardia; palpitations
		Sweating	ECG changes
Clomipramine	Dry mouth	Insomnia	Orthostatic
	Sexual	Blurred vision	hypotension/dizziness
	disturbances	Constipation	Tachycardia; palpitations
		Sweating	ECG changes
		Tremor	GI distress
			Weight gain (over 6 kg)
Imipramine	Dry mouth	Drowsiness; sedation	Sweating
	Orthostatic	Insomnia	Delayed micturition
	hypotension/dizziness	Excitement; hypomania	Tremor
		Headache	Tachycardia; palpitations
		Asthenia; fatigue	ECG changes
		Blurred vision	GI distress
		Constipation	Weight gain (over 6 kg)
Desipramine	None	Blurred vision	Delayed micturition
		Dry mouth	Tachycardia; palpitations
		Constipation	
Nortriptyline	None	Disorientation/confusion	Constipation
		Asthenia; fatigue	Tremor
		Dry mouth	

ECG, electrocardiogram; GI, gastrointestinal.

The selective serotonin reuptake inhibitors (SSRIs)

A major advantage of this class of antidepressants is its simple once-daily dosing regimen. For many patients the starting dose is the effective dose for both acute and maintenance therapies. When required, dose increments can be made without altering the once-daily dosing schedule (Table 6.5).

Gastrointestinal (GI) side-effects, especially nausea, are common, particularly during the first one to two weeks of SSRI treatment (Table 6.6). High rates of sexual dysfunction are reported on direct questioning but these rates are probably similar to the older antidepressants.

Dual-action antidepressants

Venlafaxine and duloxetine inhibit both 5HT and NE reuptake, while mirtazapine acts on both systems through indirect noradrenergic mechanisms. Nefazodone has weak noradrenergic effects as well as $5HT_2$ and 5HT transporter blockade. However, it was withdrawn in 2003 due to hepatotoxicity reports. Bupropion has dual-uptake blocking actions on the dopamineric and noradrenergic systems (Table 6.7).

Because of their diverse mechanisms of action, agents in this class have different side-effect profiles e.g. bupropion with dopaminergic effects

Table 6.5 Dosing of SSRIs

Drug	Dosage adjustment (mg)		
	Starting[1]	Usual[2]	High[3]
Citalopram	10-20	20-40	60
Escitalopram	10	10-20	30
Fluoxetine	10-20	20-40	60-80
Fluvoxamine	50-100	150-200	400
Paroxetine	10-20	20-40	60
Sertraline	25-50	50-100	150-200

1. Lower starting dose indicated with previous sensitivity to side-effects or with polypharmacy; often applies to elderly patients.
2. For SSRIs, upper starting dose may be usual dose, e.g. fluoxetine 20 mg, paroxetine 20 mg or sertraline 50 mg, otherwise increments every 5-7 days.
3. Higher doses often exceed recommended upper limits in formularies; these doses should be used with caution.

Table 6.6 Frequently reported side-effects across SSRIs[1]

Antidepressant	≥ 30%	Incidence of side-effects ≥ 10%	
Citalopram Escitalopram[2]	None	Drowsiness; sedation Insomnia Headache Asthenia; fatigue Dry mouth	Sweating Tremor GI distress Sexual disturbances
Fluoxetine	Sexual disturbances	Drowsiness; sedation Insomnia Disorientation/confusion Headache Asthenia; fatigue	Dry mouth Tremor Orthostatic hypotension/dizziness GI distress
Fluvoxamine	GI distress Sexual disturbances	Drowsiness; sedation Insomnia Excitement; hypomania Headache Asthenia; fatigue	Dry mouth Constipation Sweating Tremor
Paroxetine	Sexual disturbances	Drowsiness; sedation Insomnia Headache Asthenia; fatigue Dry mouth Constipation	Sweating Tremor Orthostatic hypotension/dizziness GI distress
Sertraline	GI distress Sexual disturbances	Drowsiness; sedation Insomnia Excitement; hypomania Headache	Dry mouth Tremor Orthostatic hypotension/dizziness

1. Adapted from Clinical guidelines for the treatment of depressive disorders: IV Medications and other biological treatments, Can J Psychiatry 2001.
2. Escitalopram is the stereoisomer of citalopram – comparable side-effects to citalopram have been reported.
GI, gastrointestinal.

tends to be alerting and if taken at night would be likely to increase insomnia. On the other hand, trazodone, nefazodone and mirtazapine, because of their $5HT_2$ receptor-blocking properties usually improve sleep (Table 6.8).

Table 6.7 Dosing of dual-action agents

Drug	Dosage adjustment (mg)		
	Starting[1]	Usual	High[2]
Bupropion (Bupropion SR)	75	150-300	375-450
Duloxetine	60	60-120	120
Mirtazapine	30	30-45	60
Trazodone	150-200	300-400	600
Venlafaxine (Venlafaxine XR)	37.5-75	112.5-225	300-375

1. Lower starting dose indicated with previous sensitivity to side-effects or with polypharmacy; often applies to elderly patients.
2. Higher doses often exceed recommended upper limits in formularies; these doses should be used with caution.

Sexual dysfunction across antidepressant classes

Drug-induced sexual dysfunction appears to be more common in men than women, although baseline levels of sexual dysfunction are higher in untreated depressed women than men. Reporting rates are low in studies that rely on self-report and are higher when specific questions are asked about desire, arousal, orgasm and overall satisfaction. Rates of sexual dysfunction are as high or higher with TCAs and MAOIs (this issue was usually overlooked in the presence of multiple other side-effects) compared to SSRI and dual-action antidepressants (Table 6.9).

When structured questionnaires are used to evaluate sexual dysfunction, 30–50% of patients who are treated with SSRIs or venlafaxine (comparable duloxetine data are not yet available) report impairment of desire and orgasm on SSRIs, while bupropion, nefazodone and moclobemide cause significantly less dysfunction. Mirtazapine also appears to be relatively free of sexual side-effects. A potential advantage of the tendency for SSRIs to delay ejaculation has been demonstrated in the treatment of premature ejaculation.

Weight gain across antidepressant classes

Until recently, weight change was not emphasized as an important outcome measure in antidepressant studies, although the tendency for TCA and MAOI agents to cause substantial weight gain has been recognized for many years.

Table 6.8 Frequently reported side-effects across dual-action agents

Antidepressant	≥ 30%	Incidence of side-effects	≥ 10%
Bupropion	None	Insomnia Excitement; hypomania Headache Dry mouth Blurred vision	Constipation Sweating Tremor GI distress
Duloxetine	GI distress	Drowsiness; sedation Insomnia Dry mouth	Constipation Orthostatic hypotension/dizziness
Mirtazapine	Drowsiness; sedation Dry mouth Weight gain (over 6 kg)	Asthenia; fatigue Blurred vision	Constipation
Trazodone	Drowsiness; sedation	Asthenia; fatigue Dry mouth	Orthostatic hypotension/dizziness GI distress
Venlafaxine	GI distress Sexual disturbances	Drowsiness; sedation Insomnia Excitement; hypomania Headache Asthenia; fatigue	Dry mouth Constipation Sweating Orthostatic hypotension/dizziness

GI, gastrointestinal.

It is estimated that treatment with some TCAs may produce a weight gain of approximately 1 kg per month.

SSRIs are frequently associated with modest reductions in weight during the acute phase of treatment, although there is some evidence that weight gain may occur during SSRI maintenance treatment. Moclobemide, nefazodone and bupropion SR do not appear to cause weight gain and for some patients may be associated with weight reduction. Short-term trials suggest that venlafaxine is weight neutral; however, there is an absence of controlled data on long-term weight change.

Table 6.9 Frequency of sexual dysfunction during antidepressant treatment (Level 2)

| | Incidence of sexual dysfunction | |
< 10%	10-30%	> 30%
Bupropion	Citalopram	Fluoxetine
Mirtazapine	Duloxetine	Fluvoxamine
Moclobemide	Venlafaxine	Paroxetine
		Sertraline

Among the currently available SSRI and dual-action agents, mirtazapine is most likely to be associated with weight gain during acute treatment. This reflects both histaminergic and $5HT_{2C}$ receptor antagonist properties. During maintenance treatment with mirtazapine, patients who have not experienced weight gain in the acute phase are unlikely to start gaining weight and those patients who initially gained weight are likely to maintain a plateau after the first few months of treatment (Table 6.10).

Dropout rates

Discontinuation rates in the 15–30% range are typical during acute treatment and are significantly higher in patients who receive TCAs compared

Table 6.10 Conclusions about weight gain during antidepressant treatment

Conclusions	Evidence
Acute phase	
Weight neutral	
SSRIs; bupropion; moclobemide; venlafaxine	Level 2
Weight gain	
Mirtazapine results in weight gain of 7% or more in up to 14% of patients	Level 2
TCAs cause weight gain in a significant proportion of patients	Level 2
Maintenance phase	
Data on weight change with maintenance treatment are inconclusive	
Low rates of weight gain (< 10%) are reported with bupropion, and moclobemide	Level 2

with SSRIs. Discontinuation rates are also likely to be higher in natural practice compared with clinical trials.

Potential for drug–drug interactions

Most antidepressants are metabolized by one or more of the cytochrome P450 (CYP) hepatic isoenzymes. Pharmacokinetic interactions may occur when an antidepressant or other concomitant medication also acts as an inhibitor or inducer of one or more of these isoenzymes (Tables 6.11 and 6.12). Among SSRIs, fluvoxamine is a potent inhibitor of CYP1A2 and CYP2C19, fluoxetine and fluvoxamine are potent CYP2C9 inhibitors, fluoxetine and paroxetine potently inhibit CYP2D6, while nefazodone is the most potent inhibitor of CYP3A4. In general, dual-action agents are less likely to inhibit metabolism of other agents; the clinical significance of duloxetine's 2D6 inhibition awaits further evaluation.

Protein binding may also influence the potential for drug interactions. When highly protein-bound drugs are displaced, there is a greater increase in the amount of unbound drug in plasma compared with a drug that has low protein binding. This is particularly a problem with the anticoagulant warfarin because dangerous alterations in clotting time can result. Among currently available antidepressants, most are at least 80% protein bound and many are over 90%; venlafaxine has the lowest degree of protein binding (30%) and would be least affected by competitive displacement.

Table 6.11 Pharmacokinetics of SSRIs

Medication	Biotransformation pathways	Half-life	Protein binding (%)
Citalopram and escitalopram	Demethylation in two steps involves CYP2C19, 2D6 and 3A4	37 hours	80
Fluoxetine	Demethylation involves CYP2D6	4–6 days	95
Fluvoxamine	Demethylation and deamination involves CYP2D6 and 1A2	17–22 hours	80
Paroxetine	Oxidation and demethylation involves CYP2D6	24 hours	95
Sertraline	Demethylation involves CYP3A4	25–26 hours	98

Table 6.12 Pharmacokinetics of dual-action agents

Medication	Biotransformation pathways	Half-life	Protein binding
Bupropion SR	Hydroxylation involves CYP2B6	21 hours	84% (parent)
Duloxetine	Oxidation (involves CYP2D6 and 1A2), methylation and conjugation (sulfate and glucuronide)	9-19 hours	>95% (parent); no active metabolite
Mirtazapine	Demethylation and hydroxylation involve CYP2D6, 1A2 and 3A4	20-40 hours (parent)	85% (parent)
Venlafaxine IR/XR	O-desmethylation involves CYP2D6 and others	5-7 hours (parent) 11-13 hours (ODV)	27% (parent) 30% (ODV)

mCPP = m-Chlorophenylpiperazine; ODV = O-desmethylvenlafaxine.

Safety in overdose

Particularly in countries where TCA prescriptions remain high, lethality following overdose continues to be an important concern. Among TCAs and MAOIs, desipramine and tranylcypromine have been the most lethal; however, these uncontrolled retrospective reports do not take into account prior psychiatric history, including suicidality or severity of depression.

Antidepressant discontinuation

Unfortunately, there are no consistent, evidence-based biological markers to predict recurrence, although some demographic and clinical parameters have been identified as risk factors (see Chapter 2). At the end of two years, patient and physician should confer about stopping medication. The decision reflects a balance between the benefits (preventing recurrence) and the risks (side-effects, cost and inconvenience) of staying on medications or discontinuing medication and monitoring for recurrence.

Table 6.13 Conclusions about antidepressant discontinuation

Conclusions	Evidence
• There is a modest but clinically significant difference in favour of SSRIs over TCAs.	Level 1
• There is insufficient evidence to report on novel antidepressants compared to other agents.	
• Antidepressants should be tapered slowly to avoid discontinuation symptoms.	Level 3

If the decision is made to discontinue the antidepressant, patients should be educated about prodromal symptoms that might signal impending recurrence. These will tend to be specific to each individual and may include typical symptoms such as alterations in sleep and appetite, lowering of mood or more idiosyncratic changes such as increased sensitivity to emotional films and writings. These may be preceded by periods of life stress and patients should be warned to be more vigilant about their mood when under stress.

Furthermore, when the antidepressant is discontinued it should be gradually tapered to avoid discontinuation symptoms. Some antidepressants are more likely to produce discontinuation emergent symptoms than others, particularly when they are rapidly discontinued from usual or above average therapeutic doses. Among the newer agents, paroxetine and venlafaxine are most likely to produce such symptoms, probably because their short half-lives lead to faster falls in brain levels. Tapering, and in some cases substituting one or two doses of fluoxetine, will prevent or alleviate these symptoms (Table 6.13).

Conclusions

There are still limitations associated with antidepressants in all classes. Clinicians are advised to have a working knowledge of standard dosing, side-effect and safety profiles as well as drug interactions and discontinuation effects for antidepressants across each of the main classes.

Bibliography

Bauer M, Bschor T, Kunz D *et al.* Double-blind, placebo-controlled trial of the use of lithium to augment antidepressant medication in continuation treatment of unipolar major depression. *Am J Psychiatry* 2000; **157**: 1429–35.

Bezchlibnyk-Butler KZ, Jeffries JJ. *Clinical Handbook of Psychotropic Drugs*, 10th edn. Toronto: Hogrefe & Huber, 2000.

Buckley NA, McManus PR. Fatal toxicity of serotoninergic and other antidepressant drugs: analysis of United Kingdom mortality data. *BMJ* 2002; **325** (7376): 1332–3.

Clayton AH, Pradko JF, Croft HA *et al*. Prevalence of sexual dysfunction among newer antidepressants. *J Clin Psychiatry* 2002; **63**: 357–66.

Dewan MJ, Anand VS. Evaluating the tolerability of the newer antidepressants. *J Nerv Ment Dis* 1999; **187**: 96–101.

Fulton B, Benfield P. Moclobemide: an update of its pharmacological properties and therapeutic use. *Drugs* 1996; **52**: 450–74.

Furukawa TA, McGuire H, Barbui C. Meta-analysis of effects and side-effects of low dosage tricyclic antidepressants in depression: systematic review. *BMJ* 2002; **325** (7371): 991.

Gregorian RS, Golden KA, Bahce A *et al*. Antidepressant-induced sexual dysfunction. *Ann Pharmacother* 2002; **36**: 1577–89.

Hemeryck A, Belpaire FM. Selective serotonin reuptake inhibitors and cytochrome P-450 mediated drug–drug interactions: an update. *Curr Drug Metab* 2002; **3**: 13–37.

Kennedy SH, Eisfeld BS, Dickens SE *et al*. Antidepressant-induced sexual dysfunction during treatment with moclobemide, paroxetine, sertraline, and venlafaxine. *J Clin Psychiatry* 2000; **61**: 276–81.

Kennedy SH, Lam RW, Cohen NL, Ravindran AV, the CANMAT Depression Work Group. Clinical guidelines for the treatment of depressive disorders. IV. Medications and other biological treatments. *Can J Psychiatry* 2001; **46** (Suppl. 1): 38S–58S.

Kennedy SH, Holt A, Baker GB. Monoamine oxidase inhibitors. In: Sadock BJ, Sadock VA (eds), *Comprehensive Textbook of Psychiatry*, 8th edn. Baltimore: Lippincott, Williams and Wilkins, 2003.

Kent JM. SNaRIs, NaSSAs, and NaRIs: new agents for the treatment of depression. *Lancet* 2000; **355** (9207): 911–98.

Nutt DJ. Tolerability and safety aspects of mirtazapine. *Hum Psychopharmacol* 2002; **17** (Suppl. 1): S37–S41.

Rosenbaum JF, Fava M, Hoog SL *et al*. Selective serotonin reuptake inhibitor discontinuation syndrome: a randomized clinical trial. *Biol Psychiatry* 1998; **44**: 77–87.

Sussman N, Ginsberg DL. Weight effects of nefazodone, bupropion, mirtazapine, and venlafaxine: a review of available evidence. *Primary Psychiatry* 2000; **7**: 33–48.

Vanderkooy JD, Kennedy SH, Bagby RM. Antidepressant side-effects in depression patients treated in a naturalistic setting: a study of bupropion, moclobemide, paroxetine, sertraline, and venlafaxine. *Can J Psychiatry* 2002; **47**: 174–80.

Zajecka J, Tracy KA, Mitchell S. Discontinuation symptoms after treatment with serotonin reuptake inhibitors: a literature review. *J Clin Psychiatry* 1997; **58**: 291–7.

Chapter 7

Electroconvulsive therapy and other physical treatments

Electroconvulsive therapy

Despite much misinformed criticism over the past two decades, electroconvulsive therapy (ECT) remains a vital tool in the therapy of depression. It appears to have similar but faster and more marked effects than antidepressant drugs as well as a plausible rationale for activity. ECT seems to stimulate amine function in a progressive fashion starting with dopamine (DA) then norepinephrine (NE) and finally serotonin (5HT) (Figure 7.1). These neurochemical changes and sequential alterations in second messengers and growth factors probably underline the mechanism of action of ECT to ameliorate the many symptoms of depression.

Efficacy

Among currently available physical treatments for depression, ECT is the most established and most effective. Response rates of 60–80% are reported in the treatment of major depressive disorder (MDD) although randomized controlled trials involving ECT have methodological limitations. In particular, there are very few direct comparisons between ECT and selective serotonin reuptake inhibitor (SSRI) or dual-action antidepressants.

There is evidence to suggest that response rates to ECT are higher in elderly patients compared with middle life patients. This means it is frequently used as a first choice in elderly depressed patients, particularly those experiencing psychotic or melancholic symptoms. It has been suggested that patients who are resistant to antidepressants have both a lower response rate

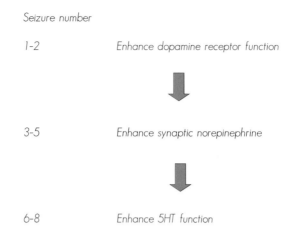

Seizure number

1-2   *Enhance dopamine receptor function*

3-5   *Enhance synaptic norepinephrine*

6-8   *Enhance 5HT function*

Figure 7.1 Proposed sequential neurotransmitter mechanisms following ECT.

to ECT and a higher relapse rate within six months. However, naturalistic studies do not show a relationship between antidepressant refractoriness and clinical outcome. ECT should be considered in the following circumstances:

- Acute suicidal ideation
- Psychotic features (delusional depression)
- Treatment-resistant depression
- Repeated medication intolerance
- Rapidly deteriorating physical status (food/fluid refusal)
- Prior favorable response.

Treatment parameters

During the acute-treatment phase, ECT should be administered two or three times weekly for up to six weeks and a typical course is 6–20 treatments. A less frequent schedule may minimize some of the immediate cognitive side-effects of ECT but response is slower.

Electrode placement may be unilateral (UL) to the nondominant hemisphere or bilateral (BL). Patients who receive UL-ECT usually experience less short-term impairment of memory or language. However, it can be harder to achieve an adequate duration of seizure, making it especially important to optimize the electrical dose relative to the seizure threshold at the first treatment. Individual assessment of seizure threshold is critical because there is at least a 12-fold range in seizure threshold among patients.

The effectiveness of ECT depends on both duration and intensity of seizures. Seizures should last at least 25 seconds, should be monitored visually and if possible by EEG. Accurate visual monitoring is best done using a blood pressure cuff to exclude muscle relaxant from one arm, so that muscle contractions can be seen. Recommendations to manage inadequate seizure activity are provided in the following list:

- Increase the electrical charge
- Discontinue any drugs that raise seizure threshold, e.g. benzodiazepines; valproic acid; carbamazepine
- Use a seizure threshold-lowering agent such as caffeine or doxapram
- Switch from unilateral to bilateral placements.

Compared with bilateral electrode placement, unilateral placement on the nondominant hemisphere at a suprathreshold dose produces fewer immediate and persistent cognitive side-effects, without compromising treatment efficacy. An electrical dose of three to six times the seizure threshold is required for unilateral electrode placement to have the same efficacy as bilateral ECT. Equipment should be adequately powered to deliver these suprathreshold doses.

With fewer hospital beds for psychiatric patients and growing pressures to reduce length of stay in inpatient units, ECT is being increasingly used on an ambulatory or outpatient basis.

Adverse effects

ECT is a safe procedure. Mortality and morbidity rates are extremely low in the modern era, approximating to the risk of general anesthesia. Apart from raised intracranial pressure, there are no absolute contraindications. Careful preanesthetic examination is essential, particularly for patients who have additional risk factors, including myocardial ischemia, cardiac arrhythmias, pacemakers or an abdominal aneurysm. Mortality associated with ECT is estimated to be 0.2 per 100 000 treatments and is most often related to cardiovascular anaesthetic complications. The adverse event rate associated with ECT is around 0.4%. Adverse events can include musculoskeletal or dental injuries, superficial skin burns, oral lacerations and persistent myalgia (secondary to the muscle relaxant). Nausea, headaches and muscle aches are common posttreatment events, which can be treated with anti-emetics or analgesics.

The cognitive side-effects associated with ECT are well documented. Objective memory testing shows a marked improvement compared to the profound impairment associated with depression but there is evidence of residual retrograde amnesia. This lessens with time, so that no cognitive deficits are apparent six months after treatment, although there may be persistent lacunae of memory deficits for events occurring around the time of the ECT. Subjective memory complaints include immediate and often persistent (at least two months) deficits in some aspects of autobiographical memory (mostly impersonal memories such as public events).

BL-ECT is associated with greater cognitive side-effects than UL-ECT, as are electrical dosages above threshold levels, more frequent administration (three times rather than twice a week) and persistence of depressed mood state.

Maintenance ECT is less likely to cause cognitive side-effects, possibly due to the longer time interval between treatments. There is no credible evidence that ECT causes any form of structural brain damage; in fact electroshock has been shown to promote neurogenesis in animal studies and prospective neuroimaging studies using CT or MRI techniques show no structural changes in the brain after ECT.

ECT in combination with antidepressant medication

There is very little evidence to suggest that combining antidepressants with ECT improves the response. When patients are receiving ECT, they have usually failed antidepressant treatment, so it does not make sense to continue the same medication. Starting a new medication during ECT causes clinical confusion about both efficacy and side-effects. Also, there is no evidence that starting an antidepressant concurrently with ECT has any effect on outcome, compared to starting medication after the last ECT session. It has also been reported that in some cases antidepressant drugs, including SSRIs, may prolong seizure duration.

There are claims that concurrent lithium therapy is responsible for delirium or prolonged confusion after ECT. For this reason most ECT protocols require discontinuation of lithium before initiating ECT. The use of sedatives including benzodiazepines and anticonvulsants, such as carbamazepine or valproic acid, may inhibit seizures or shorten seizure duration, therefore their use with ECT is not recommended.

Prevention of relapse following ECT

Without some form of maintenance treatment the rate of relapse following ECT is high: between 50% and 95% within six months. Predictors of relapse include medication resistance prior to ECT and greater severity of depression. Maintenance pharmacotherapy for at least one or two years is nearly always indicated to prevent relapse, although there have been very few studies to inform clinicians about treatment selection. The combination of nortriptyline and lithium was significantly more effective in reducing relapse rates following ECT compared to nortriptyline alone. Medications that were ineffective when used in an optimal fashion prior to ECT should not be used for post-ECT maintenance.

Maintenance ECT

ECT may also be used as a maintenance treatment, with titration schedules ranging from once weekly to once monthly. Suggested indications are:

- History of previous response to ECT
- Failure to remit with pharmacotherapy – non-response or intolerance
- Frequent recurrence of depressive episodes
- Recurrent delusional (psychotic) depressive episodes
- Patient preference.

Unfortunately, evidence to support the effectiveness of maintenance ECT is limited to case series and case reports. Maintenance ECT needs to be evaluated under randomized controlled conditions (Table 7.1).

Table 7.1 Recommendations for ECT

Recommendations	Evidence
• ECT is an effective treatment for major depressive disorder (MDD).	Level 1
• Indications for ECT include acute suicidal risk, severe physical deterioration, depression with psychotic features, treatment resistance to medications and patient preference.	Level 2
• Unilateral electrode placement requires suprathreshold doses of ECT for optimal results.	Level 2
• Side-effects of ECT are generally mild and frequently include transient short-term memory disturbance.	Level 2
• Maintenance ECT should be considered when maintenance pharmacotherapies have been ineffective or intolerable.	Level 3

Light therapy

Efficacy

The efficacy of light therapy for winter depression (seasonal affective disorder or SAD) has been established with response rates between 60% and 90%, while the efficacy of light therapy alone in the treatment of nonseasonal depressive disorders is more controversial. Controlled studies are limited by small sample size, short treatment duration (one to four weeks) and equivocal results. This means there is currently insufficient evidence to recommend light therapy alone for nonseasonal depression. However, its use in combination with antidepressant medications may be effective for some patients.

Treatment parameters

The fluorescent light box is the 'gold standard' light device – results of clinical trials do not support efficacy claims for head mounted devices and dawn simulators. The recommended treatment regimen requires exposure to light at an intensity of 10 000 lux for 30 minutes daily, in the early morning, as soon as possible after awakening. The light box should have an ultraviolet (UV) filter to screen out harmful UV rays. Improvement in symptoms may be apparent during the first week but full response usually takes two to four weeks.

Adverse effects

Side-effects of light therapy are:

- Eyestrain
- Headache
- Nausea
- Sedation
- Visual disturbances
- Agitation or feeling 'wired'
- Sweating
- Hypomania or mania

Side-effects are usually minimal and transient (as in the list above). They may be alleviated by a reduced dose of light; there is no evidence of ocular damage with proper use of light therapy. Nevertheless, ophthalmological assessment and monitoring are recommended if patients have ocular risk

Table 7.2 Recommendations for light therapy

Recommendations	Evidence
• Light therapy is an effective treatment for MDD with a seasonal pattern (winter depression), of mild-to-moderate severity.	Level 1
• An adequate trial of light therapy requires two to four weeks of fluorescent light at an intensity of 10 000 lux for 30 minutes each day in the early morning.	Level 2
• Patients usually need to continue daily light therapy throughout the winter and can discontinue treatment in the summer.	Level 3
• There is insufficient evidence to recommend light therapy for long-term or maintenance use.	None

factors for potential light toxicity, such as pre-existing retinal disease or are being treated with photosensitizing medications including phenothiazine antipsychotics, lithium, melatonin or St John's Wort.

Maintenance light therapy

Since most patients experience rapid recurrence of symptoms after discontinuation of light therapy it should be continued throughout the period of risk for winter depression and discontinued during the summer months (Table 7.2). There are few data on long-term or maintenance uses of light therapy for SAD or nonseasonal depression.

High frequency repeated transcranial magnetic stimulation

Efficacy

There have been encouraging results in a number of small randomized trials, comparing high frequency repeated transcranial magnetic stimulation (rTMS) to antidepressants and ECT. Although ECT was superior to rTMS in MDD patients with psychotic symptoms, nonpsychotic patients responded equally well to both treatments. The authors of a recent review concluded that while it is premature to recommend rTMS in the treatment of depression, this method deserves further investigation. This treatment, and those that follow, are summarized in Table 7.3.

Table 7.3 Recommendations for other physical treatments

Recommendations	Evidence
• High frequency rapid transcranial magnetic stimulation (rTMS) and vagal nerve stimulation (VNS) are investigational biological treatments; there is too little evidence to recommend either for general clinical use.	Level 2
• Neurosurgery for depressive disorders has limited evidence for efficacy but should be considered in the most refractory and chronic cases.	Level 3
• Sleep deprivation is an effective transient treatment for depressive disorders and may also be used to augment other treatments; response may be maintained using medications (e.g. antidepressants, lithium or pindolol) or bright light.	Level 2

Treatment parameters

rTMS involves the stimulation of cortical neurons by magnetic induction, using a brief, high-intensity magnetic field. The electrical current is rapidly turned on and off to produce a time-varying magnetic field lasting 100 to 200 microseconds. Repetitive stimulation with frequencies in the range of 1 to 20 Hz is applied over the course of about 30 minutes during a treatment session. The magnetic pulse crosses the scalp almost painlessly, causing neuronal stimulation and depolarization to a depth of about 2 cm below the surface of the brain. Mild headache and discomfort at the site of stimulation are the main side-effects.

rTMS is attractive as a potential alternative treatment to ECT because it can be conducted in outpatient settings, does not require anesthesia or sedation, has no effects on cognition and has minimal side-effects.

Combination with antidepressants

Potential clinical uses include the treatment of medication-refractory patients, perhaps in place of ECT. Because of its rapid onset of effect, it may also hasten clinical response in conjunction with antidepressants. As yet, however, there is no consensus about the optimal treatment parameters, including frequency and anatomic location of stimulation. Most of the positive results have yet to be replicated, the follow-up periods are brief and there are no long-term or maintenance studies.

Surgical treatments

Vagus nerve stimulation: efficacy and treatment parameters

Vagus nerve stimulation (VNS) is approved for the treatment of drug-refractory epilepsy and in some countries it is being investigated for treatment-resistant MDD.

An electrical wire is surgically implanted around the right vagus nerve in the neck and connected to a stimulator located in the chest wall. In an open trial, intermittent stimulation of the vagus nerve resulted in a 40% response rate in treatment-resistant patients. Unfortunately, controlled studies have yet to confirm these preliminary results.

Neurosurgery for psychiatric disorders: efficacy and parameters

Modern neurosurgery techniques involve the placement of stereotactically positioned lesions in different limbic areas of the brain. The procedures currently in use are anterior cingulotomy or capsulotomy and subcaudate tractotomy. There are no controlled studies of modern limbic surgery yet reported, although a multinational study using a noninvasive gamma knife approach is ongoing.

In several open series involving treatment-resistant patients, between 30% and 60% of patients had good or very good improvement; mortality and morbidity rates are very low. No significant behavioural or intellectual deficits, and few changes in personality, have been reported for the procedures, though epilepsy and frontal syndromes are rare complications. Neurosurgery should be considered for depressed patients with the most intractable illnesses.

Sleep deprivation

Efficacy

Total sleep deprivation (TSD) can improve depressive symptoms, sometimes dramatically. On occasion manic switches have been triggered in bipolar patients. Unfortunately, the antidepressant effect of TSD is usually transient and most patients relapse after even a brief recovery of sleep, leaving a minority (up to 15%) in sustained remission.

In an effort to prevent this rapid relapse after TSD, modified partial sleep deprivation (i.e. sleep deprivation in the second half of the night) has been evaluated with some success. Unfortunately, even partial sleep deprivation is difficult for patients to continue for more than a week, and when carried out in hospital is quite demanding on nursing staff.

Treatment parameters

Given the rather simple procedure, sleep deprivation may be considered as an alternative approach, particularly when a rapid response is required (e.g. in acutely suicidal inpatients). One protocol supported in the literature includes three total sleep deprivation periods within one week. During each 48-hour period, the patient is awake from 7 am on Day 1 to 7 pm on Day 2 (36 hours of sleep deprivation) followed by recovery sleep from 7 pm to 7 am on Day 3 (12 hours sleep). The next sleep deprivation period is repeated.

Combination and maintenance

Strategies to sustain the antidepressant effect include combining sleep deprivation with antidepressant medications, lithium, pindolol, bright light treatment and, paradoxically, tryptophan depletion. Placebo-controlled studies are obviously difficult to conduct for such a treatment but several controlled studies of sleep deprivation support these combined treatments. Sleep deprivation has no evidence base to recommend it as a maintenance therapy.

Bibliography

Berman RM, Narasimhan M, Sanacora G *et al*. A randomized clinical trial of repetitive transcranial magnetic stimulation in the treatment of major depression. *Biol Psychiatry* 2000; **47**: 332–7.

Bourgon LN, Kellner CH. Relapse of depression after ECT: a review. *J ECT* 2000; **16**: 19–31.

Duman RS, Malberg J, Nakagawa S, D'Sa C. Neuronal plasticity and survival in mood disorders. *Biol Psychiatry* 2000; **48** (8): 732–9.

George M, Belmaker R. *Transcranial Magnetic Stimulation in Psychiatry*. Washington DC: American Psychiatric Press, 2000.

George MS, Nahas Z, Bohning DE *et al*. Vagus nerve stimulation therapy: a research update. *Neurology* 2002; **59** (6 Suppl. 4): S56–S61.

Giedke H, Schwarzler F. Therapeutic use of sleep deprivation in depression. *Sleep Med Rev* 2002; **6**(5): 361–77.

Janicak PG, Dowd SM, Martis B *et al*. Repetitive transcranial magnetic stimulation versus electroconvulsive therapy for major depression: preliminary results of a randomized trial. *Biol Psychiatry* 2002; **51** (8): 659–67.

Kripke DF. Light treatment for nonseasonal depression: speed, efficacy, and combined treatment. *J Affect Disord* 1998; **49**: 109–17.

Lam RW, Levitt AJ. *Canadian Consensus Guidelines for the Treatment of Seasonal Affective Disorder*. Vancouver, BC: Clinical & Academic Publishing, 1999.

Lam RW, Bartley S, Yatham LN *et al*. Clinical predictors of short-term outcome in electroconvulsive therapy. *Can J Psychiatry* 1999; **44**: 158–63.

Lee TM, Chan CC. Dose-response relationship of phototherapy for seasonal affective disorder: a meta-analysis. *Acta Psychiatr Scand* 1999; **99**: 315–23.

Lisanby SH, Maddox JH, Prudic J *et al*. The effects of electroconvulsive therapy on memory of autobiographical and public events. *Arch Gen Psychiatry* 2000; **57**: 581–90.

Malhi GS, Sachdev P. Novel physical treatments for the management of neuropsychiatric disorders. *J Psychosom Res* 2002; **53**: 709–19.

Mayur PM, Gangadhar BN, Subbakrishna DK, Janakiramaiah N. Discontinuation of antidepressant drugs during electroconvulsive therapy: a controlled study. *J Affect Disord* 2000; **58**: 37–41.

Nutt DJ, Glue P. The neurobiology of ECT: animal studies. In: Caffey CE (ed.) *ECT: From Research to Clinical Practice*. Washington DC: American Psychiatric Association, 2000, pp 241–65.

Potokar J, Wilson SJ, Nutt DJ. Do SSRIs prolong seizure duration during ECT? *Int J Psychiatry Clin Practice* 1997; **1** (4): 277–80.

Rabheru K, Persad E. A review of continuation and maintenance electroconvulsive therapy. *Can J Psychiatry* 1997; **42**: 476–84.

Rush AJ, George MS, Sackeim HA *et al*. Vagus nerve stimulation (VNS) for treatment-resistant depressions: a multicenter study. *Biol Psychiatry* 2000; **47**: 276–86.

Sackeim HA, Haskett RF, Mulsant BH *et al*. Continuation pharmacotherapy in the prevention of relapse following electroconvulsive therapy: a randomized controlled trial. *JAMA* 2001; **285**: 1299–307.

Sackeim HA, Prudic J, Devanand DP *et al*. A prospective, randomized, double-blind comparison of bilateral and right unilateral electroconvulsive therapy at different stimulus intensities. *Arch Gen Psychiatry* 2000; **57**: 425–34.

Tew JD Jr, Mulsant BH, Haskett RF *et al*. Acute efficacy of ECT in the treatment of major depression in the old-old. *Am J Psychiatry* 1999; **156**: 1865–70.

UK ECT Review Group. Efficacy and safety of electroconvulsive therapy in depressive disorders: a systematic review and meta-analysis. *Lancet* 2003; **361** (9360): 799–808.

Wirz-Justice A, van den Hoofdakker RH. Sleep deprivation in depression: what do we know, where do we go? *Biol Psychiatry* 1999; **46**: 445–53.

Chapter 8

Complementary therapies

Introduction

Worldwide consumer interest in self-administered herbal preparations and supplemental products has grown exponentially in the past decade. In almost every case this has occurred with only anecdotal evidence to support the effectiveness of these products, with only limited knowledge about established dosing regimens and amidst concerns about internal consistency in the manufacturing processes.

This chapter will consider medicines and dietary supplements as well as lifestyle interventions that are not endorsed by typical health care payers. Only studies that describe diagnostic criteria for inclusion of depressed patients and include accepted outcome measures are considered.

St John's Wort

Extracts of the plant St John's Wort (*Hypericum perforatum*) have been reported to lift mood for centuries, especially in central Europe. Since the publication of a meta-analysis in 2001 supporting the efficacy of *H. perforatum* in depression of mild-to-moderate severity, there have been at least three large trials, two in the USA and one in France, that met standards for good clinical trial design. In both US studies, *H. perforatum* was no more efficacious than placebo, although in one of these trials the active comparator agent sertraline was also no more effective than placebo. In contrast, results of the European placebo-controlled trial supported Hypericum as an effective antidepressant in mild-to-moderate depression.

Table 8.1 Side-effects and drug interactions of *Hypericum perforatum.*

Side-effects	Drug interactions
Gastrointestinal discomfort	Serotonin syndrome with SSRI
Photosensitivity	Decreased effect of warfarin and protease inhibitors due to
Fatigue	enzyme induction
Hypomania	

The dosages of *H. perforatum* used in trials ranged from 300 to 900 mg daily. Side-effects appear to be milder and less frequent than those reported with standard antidepressants. There are, however, reports of interactions between *H. perforatum* and several prescription medications, including SSRIs (Table 8.1).

Up to nine potentially active ingredients have been identified, with recent evidence suggesting that hyperforin has mild serotonin reuptake blocking effects as well as weak effects on GABA receptors. Weak monoamine oxidase inhibition has also been observed. It is likely that different preparations contain different amounts of hyperforin and other ingredients such as hypericin.

Omega-3 fatty acids and inositol

Phospholipids are the main structural elements of all internal and external neuronal membranes and contain both highly unsaturated fatty acids from the Omega-3 or Omega-6 series as well as inositol.

Dietary sources of Omega-3 essential fatty acids include cold-water fish such as salmon and halibut as well *as canola* and soya bean oils. There are suggestions that these fatty acids may have therapeutic benefits in athero-sclerotic heart disease as well as depression. Several preparations including α-linolenic acid and ethyl-eicosapentaenoate (E-EPA) are available.

Building on previous reports of phospholipid abnormalities in depressed patients, several investigators have added E-EPA to standard antidepressants in unresponsive patients and reported antidepressant benefits. There is also evidence that Omega-3 fatty acids may help to protect against relapse when added to traditional mood stabilizers in bipolar patients. Side-effects include gastrointestinal discomfort, flatulence and a malodorous 'fishy' breath.

Inositol is thought to act as a second messenger for $5HT_2$ receptors. Several small clinical trials suggest that inositol may be helpful in depression and anxiety disorders, although it has not been effective as an adjunctive agent with SSRIs. It requires large oral doses (12 g) and may cause gastrointestinal distress and fish-like odors.

S-adenosyl methione

S-adenosyl methione (SAMe) is a naturally occurring amino acid derivative that is found in all cells. It plays a role in methylation, and as a dietary supplement may increase the availability of neurotransmitters including the monoamines: 5HT, DA and NE.

In a meta-analysis of studies comparing SAMe mainly to low-dose TCAs, there was comparable antidepressant effectiveness and in several cases patients on SAMe developed mania. There are no comparisons with SSRI or dual-action antidepressants. Although SAMe has been of interest to practitioners of complementary medicine for over a decade, it has only recently emerged in the USA as a popular self-administered treatment for depression. Nausea is a relatively common side-effect.

Tryptophan

Tryptophan was withdrawn in the USA and several European countries following the outbreak of eosinophilia myalgia syndrome, which was traced to the presence of a bacterial contaminant in a single manufacturing batch of the product. It has continued to be available by prescription only in Canada where it is subject to higher levels of quality control than nonprescription health supplements.

Although there is limited evidence that tryptophan has antidepressant effects on its own, there is more evidence to support its use as an augmentation therapy in depressed patients, with evidence that it improves sleep when combined with fluoxetine. It is generally well tolerated but may cause serotonergic syndrome when used in high doses with high-dose SSRI therapy. Tryptophan in doses of 2–6 g daily is also used as a hypnotic.

Dehydroepiandrosterone

Dehydroepiandrosterone (DHEA) is a precursor of androstenodione, which is converted to estrogens and androgens. Although there are some preliminary reports of its antidepressant properties, potential adverse effects, including increased risk of prostate cancer and liver toxicity, should limit its use in depressed patients.

Exercise

Intuitively, exercise makes sense as an adjunct to virtually all forms of anti-depressant therapies. Unfortunately there are very few studies involving exercise that meet methodological standards. In one of the only controlled trials involving elderly people with depression, exercise alone was as effective as sertraline alone or the combination of both, although sertraline produced a faster onset of response. In a six-month follow-up to this study, the exercise group had a lower relapse rate than did the medication group. Including exercise in a treatment program may also help to address concerns about medication-related weight gain.

Conclusions for the therapies mentioned in this chapter are summarized in Table 8.2.

Table 8.2 Conclusions for complementary therapies

Conclusions	Evidence
St John's Wort Contradictory findings in MDD; limited support for use in mild cases of depression; drug interactions have been reported	Level 1
Omega-3 fatty acids Potential augmentation strategy	Level 2
Inositol Some evidence of antidepressant effects; use limited by large dosing requirements	Level 3
SAMe Meta-analytic comparison with low-dose TCAs suggests limited antidepressant benefit	Level 1
Tryptophan Potential antidepressant and hypnotic effects as an augmentation strategy	Level 2
DHEA Potential hazards may outweigh antidepressant benefits	Level 2
Exercise May be effective in patients with mild depression and can be used to augment first-choice treatments	Level 1

Bibliography

Hypericum Depression Trial Study Group. Effect of *Hypericum perforatum* (St John's Wort) in major depressive disorder. *JAMA* 2002; **287**: 1807–14.

Jorm AF, Christensen H, Griffiths KM, Rodgers B. Effectiveness of complementary self-help treatments for depression. *MJA* 2002; **176**: S84–S96.

Lawlor DA, Hopker SW. The effectiveness of exercise as an intervention in the management of depression: systematic review and meta-regression analysis of randomised controlled trials. *BMJ* 2001; **322**(7289): 763–7.

Lecrubier Y, Clerc G, Didi R, Kieser M. Efficacy of St. John's Wort extract WS 5570 in major depression: a double-blind, placebo-controlled trial. *Am J Psychiatry* 2002; **159**: 1361–6.

Levitan RD, Shen J-H, Jindal R *et al.* Preliminary randomized double-blind placebo-controlled trial of tryptophan combined with fluoxetine to treat major depressive disorder: antidepressant and hypnotic effects. *J Psychiatry Neurosci* 2000; **25**: 337–46.

Nemets B, Stahl Z, Belmaker RH. Addition of Omega-3 fatty acid to maintenance medication treatment for recurrent unipolar depressive disorder. *Am J Psychiatry* 2002; **159**: 477–9.

Peet M, Horrobin DF. A dose-ranging study of the effects of ethyl-eicosapentaenoate in patients with ongoing depression despite apparently adequate treatment with standard drugs. *Arch Gen Psychiatry* 2002; **59**: 913–19.

Shelton RC, Keller MB, Gelenberg A *et al.* Effectiveness of St John's Wort in major depression: a randomized controlled trial. *JAMA* 2001; **285**: 1978–86.

Wolkowitz OM, Reus VI, Keebler A *et al.* Double-blind treatment of major depression with dehydroepiandrosterone. *Am J Psychiatry* 1999; **156**: 646–9.

Chapter 9

Treatment-resistant depression

Sequential approach to managing major depressive disorder

There is no generally accepted evidence-based sequence for antidepressant interventions in patients who do not achieve remission with the first antidepressant trial. However, there is agreement on the range of interventions that should be considered. One sequence for optimization, switching, augmentation and combination strategies is suggested in Figure 9.1.

It is important to establish a timeline for each trial; if there is no evidence of a minimal or partial response after four to six weeks of treatment at a therapeutic dosage, the probability of obtaining a remission decreases progressively. The corollary to this is that even a minimal response after two weeks (e.g. 20% reduction in symptom ratings) is a significant predictor of a favourable response after six to eight weeks. In other words, clinicians should carefully assess the effectiveness of any antidepressant after four to six weeks and be prepared to optimize the dose, switch agents or apply an augmentation or combination strategy.

Optimization

All antidepressants have a minimal therapeutic dose but only some display a linear relationship between dose and response. Practically speaking, optimization usually means increasing the dose to the maximum approved dose or until limited by side-effects. Exceptions include nortriptyline, which has a limited 'window' of therapeutic efficacy, above which antidepressant effects

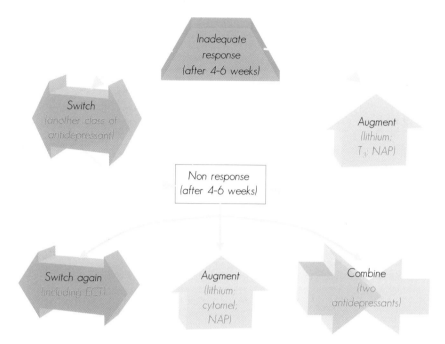

Figure 9.1 Sequential approach to poor or limited response to the initial optimized antidepressant. ECT = electroconvulsive therapy; T_3 = triiodothyronine; NAP = novel antipsychotic agent

are reduced. In contrast, selective serotonin reuptake inhibitors (SSRIs) do not show a dose–response pattern, which limits the value of obtaining plasma levels. Among the dual-action agents, venlafaxine shows most evidence of a dose–response relationship, with higher response rates at the higher dose ranges; this has been linked to the engagement of norepinephrine (NE) transporter blockade at doses of 125 mg or more. Duloxetine has yet to be evaluated at higher than recommended dose levels, while mirtazapine does not appear to offer increased effectiveness above 60 mg daily. Safety concerns about increased risk of seizure have limited the use of high-dose bupropion.

Patient differences also need to be considered. Individual variations in rates of drug metabolism may result in some patients requiring higher than usual doses, while others may require very low doses. Studies also suggest that some patients have genetically determined differences in side-effect sensitivities. Brain imaging studies of receptor or transporter occupancy may offer a clinically useful measure of maximum dosing, although these techniques are not available routinely.

If there is only partial or no response to an optimized dose of an anti-depressant, the clinician should re-evaluate diagnostic issues – in particular evidence of bipolarity, depressive subtype, comorbidity or substance abuse – and also re-evaluate treatment issues (compliance and unreported side-effects) including suicide reassessment. Basic psychoeducation and psychotherapy strategies should also be considered (see Chapter 3). Whether psychotherapy is the primary treatment or is complementary to pharmacotherapy, it may be helpful to identify one or more psychological targets for intervention (Table 9.1).

Beyond the first antidepressant

Up to 15% of patients will show no response to the first antidepressant, and perhaps 25% more will have a suboptimal response (either partial response or residual symptoms), so that up to 40% of patients will have an inadequate response. While two-thirds of these patients may respond to a second antidepressant, there remains a large proportion with 'treatment-resistant depression' (TRD). There is as yet no consensus on a definition for TRD but the most commonly used is lack of response to adequate trials of two or more antidepressants in different classes. While most studies of TRD have used this definition for eligibility, one problem is that it does not account for partial responses or clinical response with residual symptoms. It also assumes

Table 9.1 Suggested psychotherapy targets and interventions in treatment-resistant depression

Targets	Interventions
Demoralization and hopelessness	Set short-term goals
Dependency and other neurotic traits	Learn to tolerate loneliness; recognize effect on others
Inactivity/anergia	Participate in some activity
Inadequate social support	Educate the family; re-establish existing relationships
Symptom distress	Specific interventions for anxiety, insomnia and poor concentration

Adapted with permission from *Thase and Howland 1994*.

that switching medications is the first recommended strategy but this has not been systematically evaluated and may not be true in situations where there is partial response to the first antidepressant.

In two studies, these strategies were compared with different results. In one study, there were no differences between optimization (higher-dose fluoxetine), augmentation (lithium added to standard-dose fluoxetine) and combination (desipramine added to fluoxetine), although lower than usual doses were prescribed in the combination and augmentation groups. In the other study, optimization (higher-dose sertraline) was less effective than combination (mianserin added to sertraline) and placebo (added to same-dose sertraline).

Therefore, in the absence of evidence-based principles, a number of factors – including the side-effect burden of a particular medication, whether there is a partial response to the index antidepressant, potential side-effects of new treatments and previous medication history – should be used to guide the sequence of treatment selection.

Switching strategies

Antidepressants can be switched either within a medication class or to a different class. There is no evidence to support switching within the TCA class, but switching among SSRIs can be effective, particularly when the reason for switching is lack of tolerability and not lack of efficacy. However, most clinicians switch from one class of antidepressant to another (e.g. from SSRI to SNRI or TCA) when there has been no response to the first drug. Other antidepressants with distinct modes of action beyond 5HT transporter blockade (e.g. bupropion; mirtazapine; reboxetine) should also be considered if they are available. The judicious use of MAOIs should still be considered for TRD provided appropriate dietary and drug precautions are followed.

Generally, there is no need for a washout period between stopping one antidepressant and starting another. As the first antidepressant is being tapered, the new agent is added ('cross-over') but some patients may experience additive side-effects in the overlap period. For a patient who has not tolerated the first antidepressant, it may be wise to provide a washout period, allowing the side-effects to dissipate before starting a second antidepressant. It is necessary, however, to implement a two-week washout (four to five weeks for fluoxetine) before starting MAOI therapy. There is also a need to wait two weeks after discontinuing MAOI therapy before starting another antidepressant (including the switch from phenelzine to tranylcypromine).

Drug–drug interactions related to the cytochrome P450 system must also be considered during a cross-over switch. For example, when switching from fluoxetine (a long half-life SSRI that significantly inhibits CYP2D6) to desipramine (a TCA that requires this isoenzyme for metabolism), the starting dose of desipramine should be lower than usual. If problems emerge, plasma levels of desipramine should be obtained as there is significant risk for cardiotoxicity.

Augmentation and combination strategies

Technically, 'augmentation' describes adding a medication that by itself is not an antidepressant. The addition of an antidepressant at lower than usually effective doses is also considered to be an augmentation strategy, while 'combination' therapy involves the prescription of two antidepressants at therapeutic doses. However, these terms are often used interchangeably.

Table 9.2 summarizes the augmentation strategies for TRD. There is more evidence to support antidepressant augmentation with lithium and novel antipsychotic agents than with other agents. Most of the evidence with lithium and triiodothyronine augmentation involves TCAs but some studies

Table 9.2 Recommendations for augmentation strategies in treatment-resistant depression

Therapeutic choice	Recommendations	Dose	Evidence
First	Lithium	600-900 mg or to therapeutic serum levels	Level 1
	Olanzapine	5-15 mg	Level 1
Second	Risperidone and probably other novel antipsychotic agents	0.5-2 mg	Level 3
	Triiodothronine (T_3)	25-50 µg	Level 2
Third	Buspirone Lamotrigine Psychostimulants Trazodone Tryptophan	Usual doses	All Level 3
Not recommended	Pindolol	n/a	Level 1

show effectiveness of lithium with SSRIs (citalopram and fluoxetine). Lithium-induced side-effects are dose related.

There is emerging evidence that novel antipsychotic agents are effective augmentation agents for nonpsychotic MDD and TRD. Olanzapine (5–15 mg daily) in combination with fluoxetine (20–60 mg daily) was significantly more effective than either agent alone for TRD in several trials. Preliminary open-label data also support the use of risperidone (0.5–2.0 mg daily) in combination with SSRI and MAOI antidepressants.

Other augmentation strategies have been evaluated in patients who failed to respond to SSRIs. Buspirone, a partial postsynaptic $5HT_{1A}$ agonist with a metabolite that promotes NE neuron-firing, was beneficial in a number of open-label studies but a placebo-controlled trial was negative, likely because of a high placebo response rate. Pindolol, a beta-blocking drug that, in low doses, also acts as a specific antagonist of the $5HT_{1A}$ presynaptic autoreceptor was also investigated both for early onset of action and for increased response rates. However, in a large randomized study, pindolol failed to augment either an SSRI or clomipramine in refractory depression. The use of tryptophan in depression is reviewed in Chapter 8. Limited evidence exists to support its use as an augmentation agent. Although there is a long tradition of using psychostimulants to augment antidepressants, the evidence to support this is largely case based. These reports suggest they mainly reduce morning retardation. Modafinil, a new nondopaminergic stimulant, is currently being investigated for this indication. There is also anecdotal evidence to support the use of trazodone in low doses as an augmentation strategy, particularly to improve insomnia.

Combination strategies

One of the first combination antidepressant strategies to be evaluated involved an MAOI with a TCA. However, in the only controlled trial, this combination was not superior to treatment with either agent alone, and given the safety risks, it is rarely used. Since then numerous combinations have been advocated but surprisingly few have been studied in a controlled design.

Two antidepressants with complementary modes of action are often prescribed in TRD (Table 9.3). Theoretically this should enhance antidepressant effects but it may also allow one agent to offset the adverse effects of the other. For example, bupropion combined with an SSRI or venlafaxine may increase remission rates and improve sexual dysfunction. Similarly, adding mirtazapine to an SSRI or venlafaxine provides potential additional anti-

Table 9.3 Recommendations for combination strategies in treatment-resistant depression

Therapeutic choice	Recommendations	Evidence
First	SSRI + mirtazapine/mianserin	Level 2
Second	SSRI/SNRI + bupropion SR	Level 3
Third	SSRI + TCA (caution for increased serum TCA levels with some SSRIs)	Level 2
	SSRI + RIMA (reversible inhibitor of monoamine oxidase A) (caution for serotonin syndrome)	Level 3

depressant action and may also improve sleep, nausea or sexual dysfunction. Other examples of potentially additive antidepressant effects include the combination of fluoxetine and desipramine as well as moclobemide and SSRIs. The combination of fluoxetine and desipramine, however, is not recommended due to potentially dangerous kinetic interactions resulting in high plasma desipramine levels and cardiac deaths. Mianserin, like mirtazapine, has presynaptic α_2-blocking properties that indirectly enhance both noradrenergic and serotonergic transmission. This drug has been effective in combination with TCAs as well as sertraline and fluoxetine.

Generally, adding two antidepressants in combination is well tolerated but drug–drug interactions must be considered.

Conclusions

Advantages of switching from one to another antidepressant, compared to augmentation or combination strategies, include the simplicity of monotherapy and the lack of potential drug–drug interactions. Monotherapy may also, but not necessarily, have fewer side-effects and better adherence. Potential advantages of augmentation, compared to switching, include maintenance of therapeutic optimism (by not 'giving up' on a drug), avoidance of potential discontinuation symptoms, and the possibility of rapid response with some augmentation agents. Adding another agent also 'buys more time' on the initial medication and so may build on a partial response.

The benefits of combining antidepressants include the recruitment of using multiple neurochemical actions, building on a partial response and using lower doses of each agent. The drawbacks to combination antidepressant use include the possibility that a patient might simply have responded to monotherapy with the second agent, yet he or she is exposed to additional side-effects and the extra cost of a second medication.

Bibliography

Aronson R, Offman HJ, Joffe RT, Naylor CD. Triiodothyronine augmentation in the treatment of refractory depression. A meta-analysis. *Arch Gen Psychiatry* 1996; **53**: 842–8.

Barbee JG, Jamhour NJ. Lamotrigine as an augmentation agent in treatment-resistant depression. *J Clin Psychiatry* 2002; **63**: 737–41.

Bauer M, Dopfmer S. Lithium augmentation in treatment-resistant depression: meta-analysis of placebo-controlled studies. *J Clin Psychopharmacol* 1999; **19**: 427–34.

Baumann P, Nil R, Souche A *et al.* A double-blind, placebo-controlled study of citalopram with and without lithium in the treatment of therapy-resistant depressive patients: a clinical, pharmacokinetic, and pharmacogenetic investigation. *J Clin Psychopharmacol* 1996; **16**: 307–14.

DeBattista C, Solvason HB, Poirier J *et al.* A prospective trial of bupropion SR augmentation of partial and non-responders to serotonergic antidepressants. *J Clin Psychopharmacol* 2003; **23**: 27–30.

Farvolden P, Kennedy SH, Lam RW. Recent developments in the psychobiology and pharmacotherapy of depression: optimising existing treatments and novel approaches for the future. *Expert Opin Investig Drugs* 2003; **12**: 65–86.

Fava M, Alpert J, Nierenberg A *et al.* Double-blind study of high-dose fluoxetine versus lithium or desipramine augmentation of fluoxetine in partial responders and nonresponders to fluoxetine. *J Clin Psychopharmacol* 2002; **22**: 379–87.

Kennedy SH, Eisfeld BS, Meyer JH, Bagby RM. Antidepressants in clinical practice: limitations of assessment methods and drug response. *Hum Psychopharmacol* 2001; **16**: 105–14.

Kennedy SH, Lam RW, Cohen NL, Ravindran AV. Clinical guidelines for the treatment of depressive disorders. IV. Medications and other biological treatments. *Can J Psychiatry* 2001; **46** (Suppl. 1): 38S–58S.

Kennedy SH, McCann SM, Masellis M *et al.* Combining bupropion SR with venlafaxine, paroxetine, or fluoxetine: a preliminary report on pharmacokinetic, therapeutic, and sexual dysfunction effects. *J Clin Psychiatry* 2002; **63**: 181–6.

Kennedy SH, Segal ZV, Cohen NL *et al.* Lithium carbonate versus cognitive therapy as sequential combination treatment strategies in partial responders to antidepressant medication: an exploratory trial. *J Clin Psychiatry* 2003; **64**: 439–44.

Lam RW, Wan DD, Cohen NL, Kennedy SH. Combining antidepressants for treatment-resistant depression: a review. *J Clin Psychiatry* 2002; **63**: 685–93.

Licht RW, Qvitzau S. Treatment strategies in patients with major depression not responding to first-line sertraline treatment. A randomised study of extended duration of treatment, dose increase or mianserin augmentation. *Psychopharmacology (Berl)* 2002; **161** (2): 143–51.

Nierenberg AA, Farabaugh AH, Alpert JE *et al.* Timing of onset of antidepressant response with fluoxetine treatment. *Am J Psychiatry* 2000; **157**: 1423–8.

Perez V, Soler J, Puigdemont D *et al.* A double-blind, randomized, placebo-controlled trial of pindolol augmentation in depressive patients resistant to serotonin reuptake inhibitors. Grup de Recerca en Trastorns Afectius. *Arch Gen Psychiatry* 1999; **56**: 375–9.

Shelton RC, Tollefson GD, Tohen M *et al.* A novel augmentation strategy for treating resistant major depression. *Am J Psychiatry* 2001; **158**: 131–4.

Szegedi A, Muller MJ, Anghelescu I *et al.* Early improvement under mirtazapine and paroxetine predicts later stable response and remission with high sensitivity in patients with major depression. *J Clin Psychiatry* 2003; **64**: 413–20.

Thase ME, Howland R. Refractory depression: relevance of psychosocial factors and therapies. *Psychiatric Ann* 1994; **24**: 232–40.

Thase ME, Rush AJ, Howland RH *et al.* Double-blind switch study of imipramine or sertraline treatment of antidepressant-resistant chronic depression. *Arch Gen Psychiatry* 2002; **59** (3): 233–9.

Trivedi M. Algorithms in clinical psychiatry: a stepped approach toward the path to recovery. *Psychopharmacol Bull* 2002; **36** (Suppl. 2): 142–9.

Zullino D, Baumann P. Lithium augmentation in depressive patients not responding to selective serotonin reuptake inhibitors. *Pharmacopsychiatry* 2001; **34**: 119–27.

Chapter 10

Depression in women

Introduction

This chapter addresses the treatment of depressive disorders during different reproductive events in the life cycle of women (Figure 10.1).

Major depressive disorder

Gender differences in prevalence

Women are almost twice as likely to suffer from major depressive disorder (MDD) as men, beginning in early adolescence and continuing through to menopause. Atypical depression and seasonal (winter) depression occur even more frequently in women than men. Depressive episodes in women are also more recurrent, have an earlier age of onset and last longer. There are also

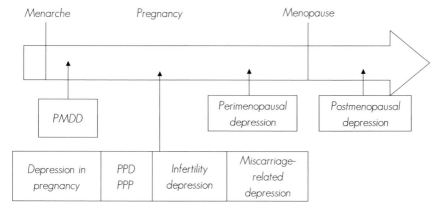

Figure 10.1 Depression and the reproductive cycle in women. (PMDD, premenstrual dysphoric disorder; PPD, postpartum depression; PPP, postpartum psychosis)

reports that depression in women is more severe, more functionally disabling and costs employers more to treat in the workplace.

Rates of comorbid psychiatric disorders also differ between men and women. Comorbid anxiety disorders are three times more prevalent in women – comorbid eating disorders and somatization disorders occur more commonly in women, whereas alcohol/substance abuse and dependence are more prevalent in men. Although borderline, histrionic and dependent personality disorders are more frequently diagnosed in women, the traditional assumption that personality disorders are more prevalent in women than men has been challenged. Rates of attempted suicide are also more prevalent in women, while completed suicide is approximately three times more prevalent in men.

The reasons for this gender difference in so many depression-related phenomena are not well understood but probably relate to a combination of physical, psychological and social factors. Women have faster rates of 5HT metabolism than men and so may be more vulnerable to reductions in the availability of the precursor amino acid L-tryptophan. Neurosteroid levels alter markedly during the menstrual cycle and in pregnancy and these can induce alterations in other neurochemicals. Social roles, especially those limiting self-effectiveness and financial autonomy, may evoke a sense of helplessness, and violence to women is more problematic due to their usually reduced ability to resist.

Gender differences in treatment response
Psychotherapy
In general, women do better than men in group therapy and in problem-solving types of individual psychotherapy, such as cognitive behavioural therapy (CBT) and interpersonal psychotherapy (IPT). One study, however, found that both men and women had similar outcomes with CBT, although among those with greater symptom severity, women were less likely to achieve remission than men.

Pharmacotherapy
Gender differences in pharmacokinetic and pharmacodynamic effects of psychotropic medications may be related to the effects of female hormones on absorption and bioavailability of medications, to differing distributions of lean/adipose body tissue, to differences in hepatic blood flow and possibly to the effects of the menstrual cycle. With comparable oral

dosing, women are likely to have higher plasma levels of antidepressant medications and experience more frequent side-effects than men. They may also be more concerned about antidepressant-induced weight gain than men and this should be taken into account when prescribing an antidepressant, especially when weight gain has been one of the features of the depression.

There is considerable controversy about the influence of menopausal status on antidepressant response. There are reports that premenopausal women respond better than postmenopausal women to selective serotonin reuptake inhibitors (SSRIs), while men and postmenopausal women respond equally well to tricyclic antidepressants (TCAs). There is also evidence that women have a better response than men to augmentation with triiodothyronine (T_3). Studies of estrogen augmentation in women with postmenopausal depression are inconclusive.

Electroconvulsive therapy (ECT)

Seventy percent of patients who receive ECT are women, which reflects the greater prevalence of depression among women. Evidence indicates that women may have lower seizure thresholds than men and that gender differences in lateralization of brain function may produce differences in cognitive side-effects of ECT (see Chapter 7 for a full discussion of ECT).

Premenstrual dysphoric disorder (PMDD)

Prevalence

The diagnosis of PMDD according to DSM-IV-TR requires five or more symptoms, for most of a 12-month time span, which start after ovulation and disappear shortly after the onset of menses (Table 10.1). They should be confirmed by at least two months of prospective ratings and cause functional impairment. Although not singled out as a core symptom, irritability is considered by many to be of particular importance. The prevalence of PMDD among women in their reproductive years is between 2% and 10%.

Psychotherapy for PMDD

To date there are no evidence-based psychotherapy studies. Cognitive therapy (CT), lifestyle therapy, stress management and attention to diet have been recommended but not evaluated.

Table 10.1 Symptoms of PMDD

Five or more symptoms must be present with at least one being either 1, 2, 3 or 4:
1. Sad, hopeless or self-deprecating
2. Tense, anxious or 'on edge'
3. Marked lability of mood with frequent tearfulness
4. Persistent irritability, anger and increased interpersonal conflicts
5. Decreased interest in usual activities
6. Difficulty concentrating
7. Fatigue, lethargy or lack of energy
8. Changes in appetite often associated with binge eating or craving
9. Hypersomnia or insomnia
10. Subjective feeling or being overwhelmed or being out of control
11. Physical symptoms such as breast tenderness or swelling, headaches, or sensations of 'bloating' or weight gain.

Pharmacotherapy for PMDD

There is strong evidence that SSRIs are effective in the treatment of PMDD. Citalopram, fluoxetine, paroxetine and sertraline have all been shown to be superior to placebo and in several cases more effective than noradrenergic antidepressants (desipramine, bupropion and maprotiline). Fluoxetine has been evaluated more frequently than the other SSRIs. The nonselective SRI clomipramine has also been shown to be effective (Table 10.2).

There is evidence to support intermittent dosing during the luteal phase only and in several studies intermittent dosing was more effective than continuous dosing.

Gonadotrophin-releasing hormone therapies may be used to suppress ovulation but are associated with substantial side-effects. Alternative therapies including St John's Wort and evening oil of primrose have not been adequately studied to allow their recommendation.

Table 10.2 Recommendations for the treatment of PMDD

Therapeutic choice	Recommendations	Evidence
First	Citalopram; fluoxetine; paroxetine; sertraline	Level 1
Second	Clomipramine	Level 2

Depression during pregnancy

Prevalence

During pregnancy, approximately 20% of women have some depressive symptomatology, and about 10% develop a major depressive episode (MDE). These rates are comparable to nonpregnant women. Risk factors include prior history of depression, younger maternal age, limited social support, living alone, greater number of children, ambivalence about pregnancy, negative life events and low socioeconomic status.

Treating depression during pregnancy

Psychotherapy

There is evidence to support the efficacy of psychotherapy for depression during pregnancy. IPT was significantly more effective than a parenting education control program in rates of maternal improvement and mother–infant interactions.

Pharmacotherapy

Concerns about potential adverse effects of antidepressants on fetal development have restricted the opportunity to carry out randomized trials. Nevertheless, data on efficacy and safety for SSRIs in almost 3000 depressed pregnant women have been published. Over 2000 of these cases involve the use of fluoxetine during pregnancy. The majority, but not all, of these studies conclude that there is no statistically significant increase in fetal abnormalities or spontaneous abortion. Similarly, no increased risk of teratogenicity was seen after exposure to citalopram, fluvoxamine, paroxetine, sertraline, or TCAs during the first trimester or throughout pregnancy.

Two large prospective surveys from the European Network of Teratology Information Services (ENTIS) and the Swedish Medical Birth Registry indicated no causal relationship between *in utero* exposure to antidepressants and adverse pregnancy outcome. In a subsequent matched comparison of infants born to mothers receiving TCAs and SSRIs compared to an unexposed comparison group, there was a decrease in gestation, birth weight and Apgar score in the infants of SSRI-treated mothers. There were no differences in the infants exposed to TCAs. Neither class was associated with congenital malformations or developmental delay. However, in a small study of infants born to women who received MAOI therapy, there was an increased risk of congenital malformations.

In another study, there was no effect on global IQ, language development or behavioural development in preschool children exposed to TCAs or fluoxetine in the first trimester or throughout pregnancy. There were also no significant differences in mood, temperament, arousal or activity levels, distractibility or behavioural problems in these groups of children.

Because pregnancy is a hypermetabolic state, it is not surprising that higher doses of antidepressants are often required, particularly in the later stages of pregnancy, to maintain adequate plasma levels and prevent recurrence of symptoms. In a retrospective review of dosing for fluoxetine, paroxetine and sertraline during pregnancy, the dose at delivery was approximately 1.8 times higher than the initial dosage, and the mean time for dose increase was 27 weeks into the pregnancy. There were no significant differences in dosage changes across SSRIs. It should be noted, however, that all SSRIs cross the placental barrier and caution is advised. Similar findings have also been reported with TCAs.

The consequences of antidepressant discontinuation during pregnancy are substantial. Up to 75% of pregnant women who discontinue antidepressant treatment experience a relapse of major depression by the end of pregnancy, with most relapses occurring in the first trimester. Inadequate antenatal care, poor nutrition, obstetric complications and postpartum depression (PPD), as well as the increased risk of exposure to tobacco, alcohol or drugs are all potential consequences of relapse. Untreated depression during pregnancy has been associated with low birth weight, neonatal distress, prematurity and a threefold increase in the risk of PPD.

The Motherisk Program is a Canadian resource center that deals specifically with the effects of medication on fetal development and other pregnancy-related concerns (www.motherisk.org). The National Women's Health Information Center at www.4woman.gov is a US website that may provide additional information.

Electroconvulsive therapy (ECT)

There are no prospective, controlled studies of ECT during pregnancy, although it is known that pregnancy may alter the seizure threshold and that fetal arrhythmias may occur as a consequence of ECT. Most of these effects can be minimized by modifying the standard ECT technique when treating pregnant patients; however, the patient's ability to understand and

Table 10.3 Recommendations for the treatment of depression during pregnancy

Therapeutic choice	Recommendations	Evidence
First	Fluoxetine	Level 1
Second	Citalopram, fluvoxamine, paroxetine, sertraline and venlafaxine	Level 2
Third	Tricyclic antidepressants (TCAs)	Level 2
	Electroconvulsive therapy (ECT)	Level 3
	Interpersonal therapy (IPT)	Level 3

evaluate the risks to both herself and her fetus should be considered in the decision to use ECT.

For a summary of the recommendations for the treatment of depression during pregnancy see Table 10.3.

Postnatal mood disorders

Prevalence

Postnatal mood disturbance occurs frequently and may be considered along a continuum of severity from 'maternity blues', a mild self-limiting disorder occurring in over 50% of new mothers in the first two weeks after delivery, to 'PPD' and 'postpartum psychosis' (PPP).

PPD, termed MDD with postpartum onset in DSM-IV-TR, requires onset within the first four weeks after delivery. However, depression occurring within three months of delivery is considered PPD by many clinicians. It affects 10% to 15% of new mothers. There are numerous risk factors associated with PPD, as follows:

1. Previous episode of PPD
2. Previous history of a mood disorder or other psychiatric disorder
3. Depressive symptoms during pregnancy
4. Family history of depression
5. Inadequate social support
6. Chronic stressors
7. Lower socioeconomic status
8. Depression and high levels of expressed emotion in one's partner.

Therefore, screening and early intervention are paramount. The Postpartum Depression Checklist and the Edinburgh Postnatal Depression Scale have been developed as diagnostic aids (Table 10.4).

Psychotherapy for PPD

Women who are at risk for PPD may benefit from counseling, enhanced social support and education prior to delivery. Counseling with a CBT focus for six sessions was as effective as fluoxetine in a small comparative trial. IPT

Table 10.4 Edinburgh Postnatal Depression Scale (EPDS)

Instructions

How are you feeling? Because you have recently had a baby, we would like to know how you are feeling now. Please circle the answer that comes closest to how you have felt in the past 7 days, not just how you feel today.

	Never/ not often	Sometimes	Often	Most of the time
1. I have been able to laugh and see the funny side of things.	3	2	1	0
2. I have looked forward with enjoyment to things.	3	2	1	0
3. I have blamed myself unnecessarily when things went wrong.	0	1	2	3
4. I have been worried and anxious for no good reason.	0	1	2	3
5. I have felt scared or panicky for no very good reason.	0	1	2	3
6. Things have been getting on top of me.	0	1	2	3
7. I have been so unhappy that I have had difficulty sleeping.	0	1	2	3
8. I have felt sad or miserable.	0	1	2	3
9. I have been so unhappy that I have been crying.	0	1	2	3
10. The thought of harming myself has occurred to me.	0	1	2	3

Adapted with permission from Cox et al. 1987.
A score of 12 or more is indicative of probable major or minor depression.

with specific modifications to help resolve marital disputes and major role transition issues after childbirth was also effective. There was also a significant benefit to involving both parents in psychoeducation compared with psychoeducation only for mothers.

Pharmacotherapy for PPD

There are some indications that antidepressant medication decreases recurrence rates for PPD. Fluoxetine, sertraline and venlafaxine have all shown efficacy.

Women with a history of PPD who began antidepressant treatment within 24 hours of delivery had a relapse rate of 6.7%, compared with a rate of 62% in women who deferred prophylaxis in one study, although nortriptyline was not superior to placebo in the prevention of recurrent PPD in another study.

Estrogen was also significantly more effective than placebo in improving symptoms in women with severe depression, although the effect was only significant after one month of treatment (onset within three months post-partum). High-dose estrogen therapy has been evaluated as a prophylactic treatment but its efficacy is mitigated by a number of considerations, such as interference with breast milk production and coadministration of anti-coagulants. In a large, naturalistic follow-up of women with PPD, some of whom requested progesterone, it was found that the relapse rate in the progesterone-treated group was 7%, compared with 67% in the nonproges-terone group. Further controlled studies are needed to confirm these impressive findings.

It should also be noted that women who suffer from bipolar illness have a high risk of relapse (35% to 50%) in the postpartum period. Lithium, given in the third trimester or 48 hours postpartum, has been shown to be prophylactic.

Recommendations for the treatment of PPD are summarized in Table 10.5.

Postpartum psychosis (PPP)

Prevalence

Postpartum psychosis (PPP) is a rare disorder occurring in two out of 1000 deliveries within the first four weeks postpartum.

Treatment

This is a psychiatric emergency that invariably requires hospitalization (on a voluntary or involuntary basis). In the majority of cases (70%), PPP is associated

Table 10.5 Recommendations for the treatment of postpartum depression

Recommendations		Evidence
Women with risk factors for postpartum depression (PPD) should be monitored closely during and following pregnancy		Level 3
If there is a history of previous PPD, antidepressant prophylaxis should be considered		Level 3
First choice	Fluoxetine	Level 2
	Interpersonal therapy (IPT)	Level 2
Second choice	CBT-focused counseling	Level 2
	Patient and partner psychoeducation as adjunctive treatment	Level 3
Third choice	Estrogen or progesterone	Level 2
	Progesterone	Level 3

with bipolar disorder and should be managed accordingly using antipsychotic, mood-stabilizing and, if warranted, antidepressant medications. ECT is also effective and can be first choice for speed of response. The risk of recurrence of psychotic episodes following a subsequent pregnancy or at other times is greater than 50%. Transdermal estrogen started 48 hours after delivery was not effective in reducing relapse in a high-risk group of women.

Pharmacotherapy and breast-feeding

There are limited data on the safety of antidepressants during breast-feeding. However, it does appear that some TCAs, MAOIs and SSRIs have no adverse effects on breast-fed infants.

Most studies of SSRIs report very low (fluoxetine) to nearly undetectable (sertraline and paroxetine) levels of the antidepressant in the nursing infant but the levels of the drug and its metabolite vary with maternal dosing. Some studies report that there is a gradient effect, with greater concentrations occurring in the later portions of breast milk (hind milk) than in the early portions (fore milk); this has been reported for paroxetine and sertraline. The use of sertraline, paroxetine, fluvoxamine and citalopram as well as venlafaxine in nursing mothers has not been associated with infant harm, although side-effects in infants have been reported. In the case of fluoxetine, at a standard dose of 20 mg daily, plasma levels were approximately

Table 10.6 Recommendations for the treatment of depression during breast-feeding

Recommendations	Evidence
Data regarding antidepressants during breast-feeding are limited; long-term developmental effects are unknown	Level 2
Current safety data do not contraindicate the use of several TCAs (amitriptyline, desipramine and nortriptyline) as well as citalopram, fluoxetine, fluvoxamine, paroxetine, sertraline and venlafaxine	Level 2

10% of maternal levels. Long-term studies, however, are not available and more studies are required to investigate possible long-term developmental effects (Table 10.6).

Depression and menopause

Prevalence

Controversy over the existence of 'involutional melancholia' has spanned several centuries. More recently, the influence of estrogen on 5HT receptors has been a topic of growing interest. There is also evidence that depressive symptoms increase around the perimenopause. Approximately 30% of women in this age group endorse symptoms associated with major depression or a primary anxiety disorder, and the association between physical symptoms and mood disorder is doubled in those women with artificial or surgically induced menopause, compared with other menstrual status groups. Given the increased likelihood of depression during the perimenopausal period it is advisable to screen women aged 45 to 55 years for depressive symptoms, particularly those who carry identified risk factors:

- History of PPD
- History of MDD
- History of PMDD
- A long perimenopausal period (>27 months)
- Surgical menopause
- Thyroid dysfunction.

Problems inherent in defining a menopause-related disorder include lack of adequately standardized diagnostic tools, variability in age and definitions of menopause, and variability in psychosocial and biological factors among women. Careful monitoring of symptomatology and endocrinological status may, however, assist in diagnosis and treatment. Considerations for treatment include whether the menopause is naturally or surgically induced, the role of hormone replacement therapy (HRT), and the nature and severity of symptoms. It is also important to determine whether a patient with a previous history of depression is having a recurrence or is suffering from menopause-related depression.

Treatment

Estrogen replacement therapy may provide some relief of vasomotor, minor cognitive and mood symptoms. In a small placebo-controlled trial involving perimenopausal women with minor and major depression, transdermal estrogen was significantly more effective than placebo. There are, however, case reports of mania occurring during estrogen treatment. This association may indicate that estrogen has a destabilizing effect in vulnerable patients. In a preliminary report, estradiol effectively treated perimenopausal depression. The use of estrogen replacement must be considered in the context of other data on long-term safety for such interventions (Table 10.7).

Most estrogen augmentation studies involved TCAs although recent studies examined estrogen augmentation of fluoxetine or sertraline, with contradictory conclusions. Treatment of women suffering from affective changes in the menopausal period is comparable to that of MDD – SSRIs can be of benefit for women on HRT, and some observations suggest that TCAs may be better tolerated and more effective than SSRI monotherapy. Mirtazapine has also proved to be an effective monotherapy. More research, however, is necessary in this area.

Table 10.7 Recommendations for the treatment of postmenopausal depression

Therapeutic choice	Recommendations	Evidence
First	Standard pharmacological or psychological treatments (in the absence of specific trials in this population)	Level 3
Second	Estrogen supplementation alone or estrogen augmentation of antidepressant	Level 2

Conclusion

It is important to recognize the influence of the reproductive system on depression in women. Clinicians should pay attention to 'at risk' stages in women's lives, diagnose depression and provide evidence-based treatments. During pregnancy and breast-feeding this often requires discussion of the risks of untreated depression compared to any medication-related concerns so that optimally informed decisions can be made.

Bibliography

Amsterdam J, Garcia-Espana F, Fawcett J *et al.* Fluoxetine efficacy in menopausal women with and without estrogen replacement. *J Affect Disord* 1999; **55**: 11–17.

Appleby L, Warner R, Whitton A, Faragher B. A controlled study of fluoxetine and cognitive-behavioural counselling in the treatment of postnatal depression. *BMJ* 1997; **314**(7085): 932–6.

Avis NE, Brambilla D, McKinlay SM, Vass K. A longitudinal analysis of the association between menopause and depression. Results from the Massachusetts Women's Health Study. *Ann Epidemiol* 1994; **4**: 214–20.

Birnbaum HG, Leong SA, Greenberg PE. The economics of women and depression: an employer's perspective. *J Affect Disord* 2003; **74**: 15–22.

Cox J, Holden J, Sagovsky R. Detection of postnatal depression. Development of the 10-item Edinburgh Postnatal Depression Scale. *Br J Psychiatry* 1987; **150**: 782–6.

Einarson A, Fatoye B, Sarkar M *et al.* Pregnancy outcome following gestational exposure to venlafaxine: a multicenter prospective controled study. *Am J Psychiatry* 2001; **158**: 1728–30.

Eriksson E, Andersch B, Ho HP *et al.* Diagnosis and treatment of premenstrual dysphoria. *J Clin Psychiatry* 2002; **63** (Suppl. 7): 16–23.

Gregoire AJ, Kumar R, Everitt B, Henderson AF, Studd JW. Transdermal oestrogen for treatment of severe postnatal depression. *Lancet* 1996; **347**: 930–3.

Grigoriadis S, Kennedy SH. Role of estrogen in the treatment of depression. *Am J Ther* 2002; **9**: 503–9.

Kessler RC, McGonagle KA, Swartz M *et al.* Sex and depression in the National Comorbidity Survey. I. Lifetime prevalence, chronicity and recurrence. *J Affect Disord* 1993; **29**: 85–96.

Kornstein SG, Schatzberg AF, Yonkers KA *et al.* Gender differences in presentation of chronic major depression. *Psychopharmacol Bull* 1995; **31**: 711–18.

Kornstein SG, Schatzberg AF, Thase ME *et al.* Gender differences in treatment response to sertraline versus imipramine in chronic depression. *Am J Psychiatry* 2000; **157**: 1445–52.

McElhatton PR, Garbis HM, Elefant E *et al*. The outcome of pregnancy in 689 women exposed to therapeutic doses of antidepressants. A collaborative study of the European Network of Teratology Information Services (ENTIS). *Reprod Toxicol* 1996; **10**(4): 285–94.

Misri S, Sivertz K. Tricyclic drugs in pregnancy and lactation: a preliminary report. *Int J Psychiatry Med* 1991; **21**: 157–71.

Newport DJ, Hostetter A, Arnold A, Stowe ZN. The treatment of postpartum depression: minimizing infant exposures. *J Clin Psychiatry* 2002; **63** (Suppl. 7): 31–44.

Nonacs R, Cohen LS. Depression during pregnancy: diagnosis and treatment options. *J Clin Psychiatry* 2002; **63** (Suppl. 7): 24–30.

Nulman I, Rovet J, Stewart DE *et al*. Neurodevelopment of children exposed in utero to antidepressant drugs. *N Engl J Med* 1997; **336**: 258–62.

O'Hara MW, Stuart S, Gorman LL, Wenzel A. Efficacy of interpersonal psychotherapy for postpartum depression. *Arch Gen Psychiatry* 2000; **57**: 1039–45.

Rabheru K. The use of electroconvulsive therapy in special patient populations. *Can J Psychiatry* 2001; **46**: 710–19.

Rasgon NL, Altshuler LL, Fairbanks LA *et al*. Estrogen replacement therapy in the treatment of major depressive disorder in perimenopausal women. *J Clin Psychiatry* 2002; **63** (Suppl. 7): 45–8.

Schneider LS, Small GW, Clary CM. Estrogen replacement therapy and antidepressant response to sertraline in older depressed women. *Am J Geriatr Psychiatry* 2001; **9**: 393–9.

Simon GE, Cunningham ML, Davis RL. Outcomes of prenatal antidepressant exposure. *Am J Psychiatry* 2002; **159**: 2055–61.

Soares CN, Poitras JR, Prouty J. Effect of reproductive hormones and selective estrogen receptor modulators on mood during menopause. *Drugs Aging* 2003; **20**: 85–100.

Spinelli MG, Endicott J. Controlled clinical trial of interpersonal psychotherapy versus parenting education program for depressed pregnant women. *Am J Psychiatry* 2003; **160**: 555–62.

Stewart DE. Antidepressant drugs during pregnancy and lactation. *Int Clin Psychopharmacol* 2000; **15** (Suppl. 3): S19–S24.

Thase ME, Reynolds CF III, Frank E *et al*. Do depressed men and women respond similarly to cognitive behavior therapy? *Am J Psychiatry* 1994; **151**: 500–5.

Wisner KL, Parry BL, Piontek CM. Clinical practice. Postpartum depression. *N Engl J Med* 2002; **347**: 194–9.

Yonkers KA, Kando JC, Cole JO, Blumenthal S. Gender differences in pharmacokinetics and pharmacodynamics of psychotropic medication [see comments]. *Am J Psychiatry* 1992; **149**: 587–95.

Chapter 11

Depression in children and adolescents

Introduction

Clinicians have very little evidence-based information to guide their choice of treatments of depression in children and adolescents. They are often forced to rely on adult-based evidence in selecting antidepressant treatments. However, recent pharmacotherapy and psychotherapy trials are beginning to evaluate the relative advantages of most treatments that have previously only been assessed in older age groups. This chapter will review the emerging literature.

Risk factors for depression in children and adolescents

Prepubertal boys and girls are equally affected by depression but the prevalence changes in teens and young adults with depression, affecting girls twice as frequently as boys. There is some evidence to suggest that girls who experience puberty much earlier than their peers are biologically and psychologically predisposed to developing depression. Early-onset major depressive disorder (MDD) is often associated with high rates of comorbid anxiety disorders including obsessive compulsive disorder (OCD). Prepubertal children who rapidly experience a major depressive episode (MDE) are also at considerable risk of developing bipolar disorder in their teens or in adulthood. Other risk factors for developing depression early in life are as follows (adapted with permission from Garland and Solomons 2002):

- Learning and developmental disorders
- Attention deficit hyperactivity disorder (ADHD)

- Anxiety disorders
- Parental separation and divorce
- Abuse, neglect, trauma or bereavement
- Chronic medical illness
- History of head injury
- First-degree relative (parent; sibling) with depression
- Drug misuse.

Psychotherapies in children and adolescents

There is good evidence to support the benefits of cognitive behavioural therapy (CBT) in 8 to 11-year-old children, although diagnostic criteria for MDD may not have been met in some studies. Similarly, adolescents (12–19 years old) have benefited significantly from individual and group CBT; also, there are trials to support interpersonal psychotherapy (IPT) in this age group. In general, these studies support the use of CBT or IPT in mild-to-moderate forms of childhood or adolescent depression. However, the efficacy of psychotherapies in severe depression and the relative effectiveness of these treatments compared to pharmacotherapies (SSRIs and dual-action agents) has yet to be established (Table 11.1).

Although there is strong evidence linking the development of depression in children to family relationships, there are no studies demonstrating that family therapy is effective in reducing symptoms of depression. It is also recognized that many children with depression grow up in healthy families.

Pharmacotherapy in children and adolescents

There have been relatively few pharmacokinetic and pharmacodynamic studies of antidepressants in children and adolescents, although metabolism usually takes place at similar or faster rates than in adults. While the 'start

Table 11.1 Recommendations for psychotherapy in children and adolescents

Therapeutic choice	Recommendations	Evidence
First	CBT for mild-to-moderate but not severe depression	Level 1
	IPT for mild-to-moderate, but not severe, depression	Level 2

low, go slow' axiom is particularly appropriate here, it also means that children may ultimately require doses that are higher than usual adult doses on a mg/kg basis. Time to response or remission may also take longer (six to eight weeks) in younger age groups compared with adults, therefore a longer than usual trial may be warranted.

Most standard antidepressant drugs have not received the approval of governmental regulatory bodies, such as the Food and Drug Administration (FDA) in the USA, for use in children because efficacy studies have not been carried out. In an attempt to correct this, the FDA requested manufacturers to carry out such trials, and results of several controlled trials evaluating antidepressant efficacy and safety in these age groups are now available.

There is enough evidence to state that TCAs should not be prescribed for the treatment of depression in children or adolescents. This is based on both repeatedly negative results and concerns about side-effects, particularly cardiac arrhythmias. MAO inhibitors are rarely prescribed in these age groups, although case series support their effectiveness in otherwise treatment-resistant patients.

SSRIs and dual-action antidepressants

Until 2003 there was evidence of efficacy for SSRIs in the treatment of childhood depression, albeit with low effect sizes. However, emerging data in 2003 regarding reports on increased suicidal ideation in children and adolescents during treatment with paroxetine and venlafaxine have led to a reconsideration about recommending SSRI or SNRI therapy in the treatment of childhood depression.

Table 11.2 Dosing of SSRIs in adolescents

Medication	Initial dose (mg)	Target dose (mg)	Dose range (mg)[1]
Citalopram	10	20	10-40
Fluoxetine	5	20	10-60
Fluvoxamine	50	200	100-300
Sertraline	50	50	50-200

1 High ends of range may exceed recommended upper limits in formularies and should be used with caution.
Adapted with permission from Kutcher 1997.

In 2003, advisory letters naming paroxetine and venlafaxine were sent to physicians warning against the use of these agents in the treatment of childhood depression. The same may be true for other antidepressants when their data become available.

Fluoxetine was significantly more effective than placebo in several trials; citalopram has also been effective (Table 11.2). There is less information about the use of dual-action antidepressants in children and adolescents (Table 11.3).

Atomoxetine is an inhibitor of the NE transporter that has recently become available to treat attention deficit/hyperactivity disorder (ADHD) in some countries including the USA. Based on its mode of action, it may also have antidepressant effects although these have not been the focus for regulatory approval. There does not appear to be the same potential for abuse with this type of agent compared to psychostimulants, presumably because dopamine release is not increased. Bupropion may be considered for chil-

Table 11.3 Dosing of dual-action antidepressants

Medication	Initial dose (mg)	Target dose (mg)	Dose range (mg)[1]
Bupropion	100	150	200-450
Mirtazapine	15	30	30-45

1. High end of range may exceed recommended upper limits in formularies and should be used with caution.
Adapted with permission from Shugart and Lopez 2002.

Table 11.4 Recommendations for pharmacotherapy of MDD in children and adolescents

Therapeutic choice	Recommendations	Evidence
First	Citalopram, fluoxetine	Level 2
Second	Fluvoxamine, sertraline	Level 3
Third	MAOIs	Level 3
Not recommended	TCAs	Level 1
	Paroxetine	Level 2
	Venlafaxine	Level 3
	Nefazodone	Level 3

dren with comorbid depression and ADHD where its dopamine and/or NE uptake blocking effects may help both syndromes (Table 11.4). Duloxetine has yet to be evaluated in younger age groups.

Maintenance therapy

There have been very few antidepressant maintenance trials in children and adolescents; sertraline was effective in one trial that lasted 20 weeks. Safety concerns about the SSRI class need to be resolved before other agents can be recommended. So far, recommendations about maintenance therapy in this population are derived from trials in adult populations although the same case can be made for children, as for adults, that the goals of therapy are to obtain and maintain remission. As in adults, discontinuation should follow a tapering regimen.

Electroconvulsive therapy (ECT) in children and adolescents

Based on limited data, the use of ECT in teenagers with depression or mania is effective and relatively well tolerated. Rates of improvement and side-effects appear comparable to those reported for adults. There are insufficient data on the use of ECT in children, and there is insufficient clinical experience with children, to inform the development of guidelines.

In practice, ECT should be reserved for the treatment of adolescents who are suffering from a treatment-resistant depressive or manic illness of such severity that the medical condition of the patient is compromised, or when the patient is at imminent risk for suicide. In such cases, it is prudent to obtain a second opinion from a psychiatrist who is not involved in the care of the patient. A comprehensive medical and psychiatric history and physical examination should also be conducted. Informed consent from both patient and legal guardian should be obtained prior to the use of ECT. Guidelines for the use of ECT in adolescence are currently under development by the American Academy of Child and Adolescent Psychiatry.

Suggestions for the use of ECT in children and adolescents:

1. **Choice of anaesthetic** Thiopentone, methohexitone and propofol (associated with shorter seizures in young people) are preferred in combination with suxamethonium as the muscle relaxant.

2. **Device and dosing** As young people have low seizure thresholds, machines that are capable of delivering low doses should be used. Brief-pulse, not sine wave, machines are preferred.

3. **Electrode position** There are no data correlating improvement with electrode placement. Unilateral placement may be as effective and may result in fewer cognitive side-effects but bilateral may be associated with a more rapid onset of improvement. Change position to unilateral if the patient becomes confused following bilateral treatment, or change from unilateral to bilateral after six to eight treatments if there is no improvement.

4. **EEG monitoring and recording seizure length** This is particularly important in this population, and prolonged seizures (>2 minutes) should be terminated with diazepam or additional general anesthetic.

5. **Number of treatments** Similar to those for adults, usual range being six to 12 treatments. The absence of any signs of improvement after six to eight treatments is an indication to discontinue.

Resistance to ECT can be defined as an absence of response after 12 treatments, of which six were bilateral. There is evidence to show that relapse rates following ECT are high in patients who are restarted on an antidepressant that was previously ineffective. Therefore, treatment with an antidepressant from a different class should be considered. The effectiveness of maintenance ECT to prevent relapse or recurrence has not been evaluated in children and adolescents (Table 11.5).

In teens, side-effects with ECT are common in the postictal period but are usually transient. Headaches occur most frequently and should be treated conservatively. When the cognitive effects of ECT were evaluated, there were no long-lasting effects on various neurocognitive functions, although short-term effects (lasting up to two months) on memory have been noted. See Chapter 7 for a more detailed discussion of ECT.

Table 11.5 Recommendations for the use of ECT in children and adolescents

Recommendations	Evidence
ECT is rarely a first- or second-choice treatment for adolescents but may be considered in depressed patients who are acutely suicidal, psychotic or treatment resistant	Level 3
There is weak evidence to support ECT use in prepubertal children	Level 4

Conclusion

Despite some evidence supporting the efficacy of fluoxetine and other SSRIs in children and adolescents, current safety concerns led to a re-evaluation of their use in this population. There is also a need to compare the relative effectiveness of antidepressants and evidence-based psychotherapies as well as to evaluate the benefits of maintenance treatments in children and adolescents.

Bibliography

Baumgartner JL, Emslie GJ, Crismon ML. Citalopram in children and adolescents with depression or anxiety. *Ann Pharmacother* 2002; **36**: 1692–7.

Birmaher B, Ryan ND, Williamson DE *et al*. Childhood and adolescent depression: a review of the past 10 years. Part I. *J Am Acad Child Adolesc Psychiatry* 1996; **35**: 1427–39.

Birmaher B, Ryan ND, Williamson DE *et al*. Childhood and adolescent depression: a review of the past 10 years. Part II. *J Am Acad Child Adolesc Psychiatry* 1996; **35**: 1575–83.

Cohen D, Taieb O, Flament M *et al*. Absence of cognitive impairment at long-term follow-up in adolescents treated with ECT for severe mood disorder. *Am J Psychiatry* 2000; **157**: 460–2.

Curry JF. Specific psychotherapies for childhood and adolescent depression. *Biol Psychiatry* 2001; **49**: 1091–100.

Daviss WB, Bentivoglio P, Racusin R *et al*. Bupropion sustained release in adolescents with comorbid attention-deficit/hyperactivity disorder and depression. *J Am Acad Child Adolesc Psychiatry* 2001; **40**: 307–14.

Emslie GJ, Walkup JT, Pliszka SR, Ernst M. Nontricyclic antidepressants: current trends in children and adolescents. *J Am Acad Child Adolesc Psychiatry* 1999; **38**: 517–28.

Emslie GJ, Heiligenstein JH, Wagner KD *et al*. Fluoxetine for acute treatment of depression in children and adolescents: a placebo-controlled, randomized clinical trial. *J Am Acad Child Adolesc Psychiatry* 2002; **41**: 1205–15.

Garland EJ, Solomons K. Early detection of depression in young and elderly people. *BC Medical Journal* 2002; **44**: 469–72.

Geller B, Reising D, Leonard HL *et al*. Critical review of tricyclic antidepressant use in children and adolescents. *J Am Acad Child Adolesc Psychiatry* 1999; **38**: 513–16.

Ghaziuddin N, King CA, Naylor MW *et al*. Electroconvulsive treatment in adolescents with pharmacotherapy-refractory depression. *J Child Adolesc Psychopharmacol* 1996; **6**: 259–71.

Goodnick PJ, Jorge CA, Hunter T, Kumar AM. Nefazodone treatment of adolescent depression: an open-label study of response and biochemistry. *Ann Clin Psychiatry* 2000; **12**: 97–100.

Harrington R, Whittaker J, Shoebridge P, Campbell F. Systematic review of efficacy of cognitive behaviour therapies in childhood and adolescent depressive disorder. *BMJ* 1998; **316**: 1559–63.

Hazell P, O' Connell D, Heathcote D *et al*. Efficacy of tricyclic drugs in treating child and adolescent depression: a meta-analysis. *BMJ* 1995; **310**: 897–901.

Keller MB, Ryan ND, Strober M *et al*. Efficacy of paroxetine in the treatment of adolescent major depression: a randomized, controlled trial. *J Am Acad Child Adolesc Psychiatry* 2001; **40**: 762–72.

Kutcher S. *Psychopharmacologic Treatment of Depressive Disorders*. Philadelphia: Saunders, 1997.

Mandoki MW, Tapia MR, Tapia MA *et al*. Venlafaxine in the treatment of children and adolescents with major depression. *Psychopharmacol Bull* 1997; **33**: 149–54.

McConville BJ, Minnery KL, Sorter MT *et al*. An open study of the effects of sertraline on adolescent major depression. *J Child Adolesc Psychopharmacol* 1996; **6**: 41–51.

Nutt DJ, Bell C, Masterson C, Short C. *Mood and Anxiety Disorders in Children and Adolescents*. London: Martin Dunitz, 2001.

Park RJ, Goodyer IM. Clinical guidelines for depressive disorders in childhood and adolescence. *Eur Child Adolesc Psychiatry* 2000; **9**: 147–61.

Shugart MA, Lopez EM. Depression in children and adolescents. When 'moodiness' merits special attention. *Postgrad Med* 2002; **112**: 53–61.

Chapter 12

Depression in late life

Introduction

Most recommendations for the treatment of mood disorders are based on evidence derived from studies of middle-life populations. Historically, this information has been applied to special populations, including the elderly, without adequate evaluation of efficacy, tolerability or safety. Yet there are age-related differences in the prevalence of depression, its clinical presentation and various aspects of treatment. The goal of this chapter is to provide a critical evalu-ation of the available data on epidemiology and treatment options as they pertain to managing depression in older adults.

The assessment and management of depression in the elderly involves several challenges. The very old are more sensitive to adverse effects of pharmacotherapy, for reasons ranging from pharmacokinetic and pharma-codynamic properties of the agents to inherent biological differences in an aging body and brain. Although several of the stereotypes about depression in this group, compared to younger adults (e.g. poorer response to treat-ment, and greater risks of chronicity), have turned out to be largely unjustified, depression in the elderly continues to cause substantial mor-bidity and mortality. Frequent medical comorbidity and the not uncom-mon need for complex multidrug regimens contribute to underdetection of mood disorders in the elderly. Reluctance to voice concerns about one's mental health or to utilize mental health services are also significant issues among the elderly, who often grew up with more stigmatized beliefs about mental illnesses and psychiatric treatments than subsequent generations. Biased assumptions persist among health care providers, who sometimes view depression as normal in the context of medical or mental impairment, resulting in an overlooked diagnosis and a missed opportunity to make a difference with treatment.

Epidemiology

The belief that depression is a natural or even inevitable consequence of aging is unfounded. Multiple studies suggest that the current and lifetime prevalences of MDD in later life (age 65 years and over) are significantly lower than at younger ages. For example, one-year prevalence rates for men and women, respectively, in the Epidemiologic Catchment Area (ECA) study were only 0.4 per 100 and 1.4 per 100, i.e. about one-third of the rates seen in younger or mid-life groups. Of course, higher rates are observed in specific treatment settings, including hospital wards and nursing homes. Patients at particular risk include those with chronic debilitating illnesses, such as dementia. There also appears to be a late-life onset variant of dysthymia that is thought to be linked to the cumulative burden of illness. As the most serious outcome of depression, suicide rates in the elderly differ from those of mid-life adults. Specifically, elderly white men have the highest suicide rates of all sociodemographic groups. There has, nevertheless, been a reduction in overall suicide rates in the elderly during the past few decades.

Treatment

Psychotherapy

Various psychotherapies have been adapted for treatment of late-life depression, including cognitive behavior therapy (CBT), interpersonal therapy (IPT) and psychodynamic psychotherapy (see Table 12.1). In one meta-analysis of time-limited psychotherapy studies, response rates were significantly higher than those observed in placebo-control groups in double-blind trials of antidepressant medications. However, as there were no direct comparisons between psychological and pharmacological treatments included in this meta-analysis, confidence in the conclusion is limited. Specifically, studies of psychotherapy and pharmacotherapy may enrol different subsamples of elderly depressed patients. Another meta-analysis found that CBT was an effective treatment as compared to waiting list or no-treatment control groups, but psychodynamic psychotherapy was not.

In the only pertinent placebo-controlled clinical trial of acute phase therapies of MDD in late life published to date (including random assignment to

Table 12.1 Recommendations for psychotherapy in late-life MDD

Therapeutic choice	Recommendations	Evidence
First	CBT and IPT for mild-to-moderate depression	Level 2

either an antidepressant or a psychotherapy), nortriptyline was significantly more effective than placebo for treatment of bereavement-related depression, whereas IPT was not. In the only relevant published placebo-controlled study of treatment of late-life dysthymia and minor depression, a study based in primary care comparing paroxetine and problem-solving therapy, results overall favored the pharmacotherapy. However, the effectiveness of this brief behavioral intervention varied markedly across clinical sites, ranging from the least to the most treatment group.

Maintenance psychotherapy

Reynolds and colleagues conducted the only long-term study evaluating the role of IPT, alone and in combination with nortriptyline, for the prevention of recurrent depression. All patients had responded to acute-phase therapy with the combination of IPT and nortriptyline and did not relapse during four months of continuation therapy. The randomized experiment thus did not begin until patients had fully recovered from the index episode of depression. Patients who were withdrawn from both medication and psychotherapy had a significantly poorer outcome than those who received one or the other of the monotherapies. In fact, nearly 90% of the patients who were both switched to a placebo and stopped psychotherapy were depressed again within two years. The greatest degree of prophylaxis was observed in the patients who received both modalities for maintenance phase therapy. The advantage of combined treatment (as compared to the monotherapies) was particularly evident among those patients aged 70 and above.

Pharmacotherapy

Antidepressant pharmacotherapy has become the cornerstone of management of depression in late life. Evidence from three meta-analyses document convincingly that antidepressant medications are effective treatments of late-life depression. The newer medications were found to be as effective as TCAs in these analyses, and generally are associated with fewer discontinuations due to severe adverse events and a lower burden of side-effects. Although not so widely used (and not available in the USA), the reversible inhibitor of monoamine oxidase A (RIMA), moclobemide, has been studied most extensively and, hence, the strongest evidence of efficacy in depressed elders.

Among the newer medications, no significant differences in efficacy across classes of antidepressants were revealed in these meta-analyses. However, results from a pooled analysis of eight RCTs suggested that therapy with the dual-action agent venlafaxine might result in higher remission rates than observed with the SSRIs. Although none of the studies included in the pooled analysis were specifically designed to examine treatment outcomes in the elderly, this finding held true across age groups. The safety and tolerability of venlafaxine has not been studied extensively in frail elders, although in a recently published trial comparing venlafaxine and sertraline, both drugs were effective and sertraline was better tolerated.

Without compelling evidence of large differences in efficacy, choice of treatment is more likely to be determined by individual physicians' experiences and differences in side-effect profiles. This is appropriate because vulnerability to the adverse effects of pharmacotherapy is a major concern when treating the elderly and concerns are not restricted to any specific antidepressant class.

Anticholinergic effects (constipation, urinary retention, dry mouth, blurred vision and cognitive impairment) and postural hypotension, which can cause falls and, secondarily, hip fractures, are of particular concern when tricyclic antidepressants (TCAs) are used to treat the elderly. For those at risk for dementia, anticholinergic effects can unmask cognitive difficulties and, in the extreme, can provoke a delirium. TCAs also have quinidine-like effects on cardiac conduction, which can worsen otherwise benign bundle branch blocks, can cause tachycardia, and have a relatively high lethality index, which makes them dangerous in overdose.

Within the TCA class, nortriptyline and desipramine are generally preferred for the treatment of depression in late life because these medications tend to cause fewer anticholinergic and antihistaminic side-effects. Blood level/treatment response relationships for TCAs have been relatively well studied, which permits somewhat greater precision in titrating to higher doses. Nevertheless, the overall side-effect burden of the secondary amine TCAs is still greater than that of the SSRIs. For example, nortriptyline has anticholinergic effects that are an order of magnitude stronger than those of paroxetine, which is the most anticholinergic of the SSRIs. Thus, even the secondary amine TCAs are now widely considered to be a second- or third-line therapy for depression in late life.

Table 12.2 Recommendations for pharmacotherapy in late-life MDD

Therapeutic choice	Recommendations	Evidence
First	Moclobemide	Level 1
	Citalopram; bupropion; escitalopram; fluvoxamine; paroxetine; sertraline; venlafaxine; mirtazapine	Level 2
Second	Fluoxetine; nortriptyline	Level 1
	Desipramine; nefazodone; trazodone	Level 2
Third	Amitriptyline; imipramine	Level 1
	Clomipramine; doxepin; maprotiline	Level 2
	Phenelzine; tranylcypromine	Level 2
Maintenance-phase treatment		
	Elderly patients should continue maintenance pharmacotherapy for at least two years	Level 1

Although the SSRIs are now generally preferred over the TCAs because of safety considerations, they generate other concerns during treatment of the frail elderly. Foremost among these are bradycardia, the syndrome of inappropriate excretion of antidiuretic hormone (SIADH) and balance difficulties, which also can cause falls. To these more serious side-effects must be added the common treatment-emergent complaints, such as sexual dysfunction, nausea, diarrhea and other gastrointestinal complaints, and insomnia. Venlafaxine (which, at lower doses, can be thought of as an SSRI) has similar side-effects, with an additional concern of elevated blood pressure at higher doses (Table 12.2).

Among the other newer antidepressants, bupropion, moclobemide, nefazodone and mirtazapine are distinguished from the SSRIs and venlafaxine by relatively low incidence of sexual side-effects. Two of these medications, nefazodone and mirtazapine, have beneficial effects on sleep, which can be a bonus for many older depressed patients, whereas bupropion and moclobemide are essentially nonsedating. Mirtazapine is the most antihistaminic of all the newer antidepressants and, as a result, can cause oversedation and weight gain. Interestingly, in one recent clinical trial response to mirtazapine was superior to response to paroxetine among patients who expressed the *APOE4* gene, which is implicated in the risk of dementia and cerebrovascular disease. Nefazodone has recently been implicated in rare cases of liver failure.

The nonselective monoamine oxidase inhibitors (MAOIs), tranylcypromine and phenelzine, are considered third-choice therapies for late-life depression, largely because of the need for dietary restrictions to avoid the so-called 'cheese effect', i.e. a hypertensive crisis triggered by ingestion of the amino acid tyramine. The MAOIs also can cause a range of troublesome side-effects, with orthostatic hypotension being the most serious in late-life patients. Nevertheless, these medications were found to be significantly more effective than the RIMA moclobemide in one meta-analysis. This analysis was not confined to studies of late-life depression, however, in which the tolerability advantage of moclobemide may have been more salient.

Pharmacokinetic factors and propensity to cause drug–drug interactions are also important when considering which newer antidepressant to prescribe. Despite approval by the US FDA for use in late-life depression, fluoxetine is not considered by many experts to be a first-line choice for late-life depression. This is because fluoxetine and its principal metabolite norfluoxetine have extremely long elimination half-lives that result in slow time to steady state and a very long time to fully wash-out the effects of the drug.

SSRIs vary in their effects on the various cytochrome P450 (CYP) isoenzymes, thus resulting in significant differences in propensity to cause drug–drug interactions (see Chapter 6). This is particularly important in elderly patients who have often been prescribed multiple medications for various comorbid physical conditions. Sertraline, citalopram and escitalopram, venlafaxine and mirtazapine are considered to have lower potential for this type of drug–drug interaction.

Maintenance pharmacotherapy

The need for maintenance treatment after successful antidepressant therapy in the elderly is at least as important as it is for younger adults. Moreover, elderly patients may be even more likely to relapse after discontinuing antidepressants, so most antidepressant responders should receive maintenance pharmacotherapy for at least two years (see Chapter 2). In a four-year outcome study of elderly patients with MDD, higher anxiety scores at time of response and longer time to treatment response were risk factors for recurrence. Therefore, treatment of residual anxiety symptoms may improve long-term treatment outcome.

There are few studies to compare the effectiveness of specific maintenance treatments in the elderly. Phenelzine was superior to nortriptyline in a placebo-controlled, one-year maintenance study of elderly patients with depression, although high drop-out rates compromised this study. There is evidence that nortriptyline is an effective maintenance pharmacotherapy, especially at higher serum levels and in combination with IPT. The TCA dothiepin has also been shown to be effective for prevention of recurrent depression in late-life depression.

Electroconvulsive therapy (ECT)

Electroconvulsive therapy (ECT) is a safe, rapidly effective and well-tolerated treatment for severe forms of MDD (see Chapter 7). It has been repeatedly shown to be a useful treatment in late-life depression, even in the presence of significant medical comorbid conditions. In some regions, ECT is used preferentially for treatment of patients who are less able to tolerate prolonged response times to pharmacotherapy (i.e. intensely suicidal patients or those who are essentially starving to death from disinterest in food). ECT is the treatment of first choice for severe depressive episodes with psychotic features and should always be considered when multiple antidepressant trials have been ineffective. Good ECT practice in the elderly requires careful pre-anesthetic medical consultation and management, minimization of concomitant pharmacotherapy that may adversely affect cognition, and vigilant monitoring of intra- and post-ECT cardiac status.

Factors influencing the choice of bilateral versus unilateral electrode placement are similar to those in younger groups, balancing the higher probability of response, fewer missed seizures (and thus fewer required exposure to anaesthetics) and longer times to relapse in bilateral placements with correspondingly greater likelihood of confusion, memory impairment or delirium.

Bibliography

American Psychiatric Association. Practice guideline for the treatment of patients with major depressive disorder (revision). *Am J Psychiatry* 2000; **157**: 1–45.

Baldwin RC, Simpson S. Treatment resistant depression in the elderly: a review of its conceptualisation, management and relationship to organic brain disease. *J Affect Disord* 1997; **46**: 163–73.

Bland RC, Newman SC, Orn H. Prevalence of psychiatric disorders in the elderly in Edmonton. *Acta Psychiatr Scand* 1988; **338**: 57–63.

Bruce ML, McNamara R. Psychiatric status among the homebound elderly: an epidemiologic perspective. *J Am Geriatr Soc* 1992; **40**: 561–6.

Bump GM, Mulsant BH, Pollock BG *et al.* Paroxetine versus nortriptyline in the continuation and maintenance treatment of depression in the elderly. *Depress Anxiety* 2001; **13**: 38–44.

Entsuah AR, Huang H, Thase ME. Response and remission rates in different subpopulations with major depressive disorder administered venlafaxine, selective serotonin reuptake inhibitors, or placebo. *J Clin Psychiatry* 2001; **62**: 869–77.

Flint AJ, Rifat SL. Maintenance treatment for recurrent depression in late life. A four-year outcome study. *Am J Geriatr Psychiatry* 2000; **8**: 112–16.

Frank E, Kupfer DJ, Perel JM *et al.* Three-year outcomes for maintenance therapies in recurrent depression. *Arch Gen Psychiatry* 1990; **47**: 1093–9.

Georgotas A, McCue RE, Cooper TB. A placebo-controlled comparison of nortriptyline and phenelzine in maintenance therapy of elderly depressed patients. *Arch Gen Psychiatry* 1989; **46**: 783–6.

Gerson S, Belin TR, Kaufman A *et al.* Pharmacological and psychological treatments for depressed older patients: a meta-analysis and overview of recent findings. *Harv Rev Psychiatry* 1999; **7**: 1–28.

Health Canada. *Suicide in Canada: Update of the Report of the Task Force on Suicide in Canada.* Health Canada, 1994.

Karel MJ, Hinrichsen G. Treatment of depression in late life: psychotherapeutic interventions. *Clin Psychol Rev* 2000; **20**: 707–29.

Kelly KG, Zisselman M. Update on electroconvulsive therapy (ECT) in older adults. *J Am Geriatr Soc* 2000; **48**: 560–6.

Lotufo-Neto F, Trivedi M, Thase ME. Meta-analysis of the reversible inhibitors of monoamine oxidase type A moclobemide and brofaromine for the treatment of depression. *Neuropsychopharmacology* 1999; **20**: 226–47.

Mittmann N, Herrmann N, Einarson TR *et al.* The efficacy, safety and tolerability of antidepressants in late life depression: a meta-analysis. *J Affect Disord* 1997; **46**: 191–217.

Mulsant BH, Pollock BG, Nebes R. A twelve-week, double-blind, randomized comparison of nortriptyline and paroxetine in older depressed inpatients and outpatients. *Am J Geriatr Psychiatry* 2001; **9**: 406–14.

NIH consensus conference. Diagnosis and treatment of depression in late life. *JAMA* 1992; **268**: 1018–24.

Regier DA, Boyd JH, Burke JD Jr *et al.* One-month prevalence of mental disorders in the United States. Based on five Epidemiologic Catchment Area sites. *Arch Gen Psychiatry* 1988; **45**: 977–86.

Reynolds CF III, Kupfer DJ. Depression and aging: a look to the future. *Psychiatr Serv* 1999; **50**: 1167–72.

Reynolds CF III, Perel JM, Frank E *et al.* Three-year outcomes of maintenance nortriptyline treatment in late-life depression: a study of two fixed plasma levels. *Am J Psychiatry* 1999; **156**: 1177–81.

Reynolds CF III, Miller MD, Pasternak RE *et al.* Treatment of bereavement-related major depressive episodes in later life: a controled study of acute and continuation treatment with nortriptyline and interpersonal psychotherapy. *Am J Psychiatry* 1999; **156**: 202–8.

Schatzberg AF, Kremer C, Rodrigues HE *et al*. Double-blind, randomized comparison of mirtazapine and paroxetine in elderly depressed patients. *Am J Geriatr Psychiatry* 2002; **10**: 541–50.

Steffens DC, Skoog I, Norton MC *et al*. Prevalence of depression and its treatment in an elderly population: the Cache County study. *Arch Gen Psychiatry* 2000; **57**: 601–7.

Tew JD Jr, Mulsant BH, Haskett RF *et al*. Acute efficacy of ECT in the treatment of major depression in the old-old. *Am J Psychiatry* 1999; **156**: 1865–70.

Williams JW Jr, Barrett J, Oxman T *et al*. Treatment of dysthymia and minor depression in primary care: a randomized controlled trial in older adults. *JAMA* 2000; **284**: 1519–26.

Chapter 13

Comorbidity: psychiatric and physical

General principles

Major depressive disorder (MDD) is such a common condition in the general population that its co-occurrence with other Axis I (psychiatric), Axis II (personality) and Axis III (physical) disorders is to be expected. However, MDD occurs much more often than would be expected by chance in many conditions (Figures 13.1 and 13.2). Clinicians can expect that many patients with MDD will have comorbid conditions. Left untreated, depression can contribute to poor compliance for treatment of

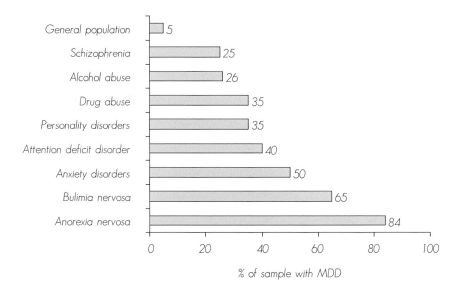

Figure 13.1 Prevalence of MDD in other Axis I disorders.

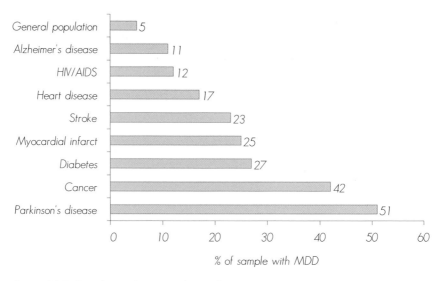

General population 5
Alzheimer's disease 11
HIV/AIDS 12
Heart disease 17
Stroke 23
Myocardial infarct 25
Diabetes 27
Cancer 42
Parkinson's disease 51

% of sample with MDD

Figure 13.2 Prevalence of MDD in chronic disease.

other medical conditions, increase length of hospital stays and increase mortality.

There are many common diagnostic and treatment issues associated with comorbid depression, regardless of the specific comorbid condition. The diagnosis of depression is often difficult to make in the presence of comorbidity. Depressive symptoms frequently accompany other illnesses and the primary condition may have symptoms that are common to MDD. For example, anxiety symptoms such as panic attacks can occur or worsen during a major depressive episode (MDE). Mood instability is a common symptom in personality disorders and can be misdiagnosed as depressive mood. In physical illnesses such as cancer, fatigue and lack of energy may not be a valid symptom of depression. In these situations, other depressive symptoms such as anhedonia, loss of interest and feelings of guilt may be helpful in making a diagnosis of comorbid MDD.

Despite the high frequency of comorbidity, there are very few controlled studies of treatment. MDD with comorbidity is usually more difficult to treat, runs a more chronic course, has greater impairment of function and is associated with greater risk of suicide compared with MDD alone. Unfortunately, most randomized controlled trials of MDD specifically exclude comorbid conditions, so results cannot be generalized to patients with comorbidity. Many studies focus only on depressive symptoms and do not include formal comorbid depressive disorders. Psychotherapeutic interventions are often targeted at the primary condition, which also may reduce secondary depressive symptoms. Similarly, studies of antidepressants for comorbidity can be complicated by other medications used in treating the primary disorder.

Not surprisingly, response and remission rates with monotherapy treatments are generally lower in patients with comorbidity. Combined treatment with pharmacotherapy and psychotherapy is usually indicated for optimal outcome. In the following sections, evidence-based treatment recommendations for both psychotherapy and pharmacotherapy are summarized for Axis I, II and III comorbidities.

Axis I and II comorbidities

Depression is frequently comorbid with other psychiatric disorders (see Figure 13.1). Among the Axis I disorders, anxiety disorders (panic disorder, generalized anxiety disorder, post-traumatic stress disorder, obsessive-compulsive disorder and social anxiety disorder) and eating disorders are most commonly associated with MDD. In some conditions, such as schizophrenia, it is very difficult to separate symptoms of depression from symptoms of the primary condition, such as negative symptoms. Specific symptom scales (such as the Calgary Depression Scale) can be useful in making an MDD diagnosis.

Personality disorders and dimensions also have a complex relationship with MDD. An estimated 30–50% of patients with MDD have a diagnosable personality disorder. There is some evidence that premorbid personality dimensions such as neuroticism confer vulnerability to MDEs. However, MDD can also result in regression and exacerbation of premorbid personality dimensions. In many studies, effective treatment of MDD leads to improvement in personality traits and patients may no longer meet criteria for a personality disorder once they have recovered from an MDE.

In the treatment of Axis I and II comorbidities, some of the same medication principles apply as for people with medical illnesses. For example, people with anxiety disorders are often hypersensitive to somatic sensations. Thus, lower initial doses and slower dose titration are helpful strategies to minimize their experience of medication side-effects. In most cases, however, full therapeutic doses are required for optimal response. Evidence-based treatments of selected Axis I and II comorbidities are summarized in Tables 13.1 and 13.2.

Table 13.1 Recommendations for the treatment of MDD with comorbid Axis I (psychiatric) disorders

Condition	Treatment choice Psychotherapy	Pharmacotherapy
Anxiety disorders	CBT [Level 3]	SSRIs and novel agents [Level 3] • panic disorder: start with lower initial doses • OCD: aim for higher doses
Substance use disorders	Motivational interviewing [Level 3]	Fluoxetine; imipramine; desipramine [Level 2] Avoid benzodiazepines [Level 3] Avoid interactions: MAOIs with opiates; SSRIs with MDMA; fluoxetine/paroxetine and codeine (opiate withdrawal); bupropion SR (increased seizure risk)
Eating disorders	CBT [Level 2]	Bulimia nervosa: fluoxetine [Level 2]; phenelzine (cautions apply) [Level 2] Anorexia nervosa: TCAs and SSRIs [Level 3]
Schizophrenia	Adjunctive CBT treats negative and positive symptoms [Level 2]	Imipramine; sertraline [Level 2] Other SSRIs [Level 3] SSRIs may help negative symptoms [Level 2] Atypical antipsychotics (olanzapine; risperidone) treat depressive symptoms in acute psychosis [Level 1] Clozapine reduces suicide events [Level 2]
Attention deficit disorder	CBT may be useful as adjunctive treatment [Level 3]	Bupropion SR [Level 3] Atomoxetine [Level 4] Fluoxetine; sertraline as adjunctive treatment for depressive symptoms only [Level 3]
Dementia	BT [Level 2]	Citalopram; fluoxetine; sertraline [Level 2] Amitriptyline; clomipramine [Level 2] ECT [Level 3]

SSRIs, selective serotonin reuptake inhibitors; OCD, obsessive compulsive disorder; MAOIs, monoamine oxidase inhibitors; CBT, cognitive behaviour therapy; BT, behaviour therapy; TCA, tricylic antidepressant; ECT, electroconvulsive therapy; MDMA, Ecstasy.

Axis III comorbidity

Depression is common and increasingly recognized as an important risk factor in the mortality and functional impairment of patients with comorbid physical illness (see Figure 13.2). There is particular interest in the relationship

Table 13.2 Recommendations for the treatment of MDD comorbid with Axis II (personality) disorders

Recommendations	Evidence
Psychotherapy	
Combined psychotherapy and pharmacotherapy may have superior outcomes	Level 3
The combination of cognitive behavioural analysis system of psychotherapy (CBASP) and nefazodone was particularly effective in a group of patients with 'chronic depression' many of whom met criteria for Axis II disorders	Level 2
Dialectical behavioural therapy is beneficial for mood symptoms associated with borderline personality	Level 2
Pharmacotherapy	
Fluoxetine (in borderline personality)	Level 3
Monoamine oxidase inhibitors (MAOIs)	Level 3
Olanzapine and risperidone (as adjunctive treatment)	Level 3

between cardiovascular disease and depression. Depression is a significant risk factor for developing coronary artery disease (CAD) and depressed patients are four times as likely to have a myocardial infarction (MI). Depression is also associated with increased mortality in patients with CAD, possibly due to alterations in the hypothalamic–pituitary adrenal axis or to decreased heart rate variability. In the first six months after an MI, there is a three- to four-fold increase in mortality among those patients with MDD, which makes it second only to heart failure as a poor prognostic indicator.

Despite the high prevalence and importance of depression in physical illness, there are very few randomized controlled trials of medically ill patients with defined comorbid depression. In contrast, there are numerous studies of psychological treatment for cancer. While several studies have shown reductions in depressive and anxiety symptoms with CBT and other treatments, none has specifically examined patients with a comorbid diagnosis of MDD. Similarly, there is sparse information on antidepressants in cancer with comorbid depression.

A recent exception is the SADHART study where sertraline was compared with placebo in the treatment of MDD post-MI. Although the antidepressant did not significantly reduce mortality or other cardiac events it was effective in reducing symptoms of depression and overall showed a better outcome on a range of cardiovascular system measures than placebo, showing it was safe to use in this group.

Antidepressants, however, are effective treatments in patients with MDD and general medical illnesses. A systematic review conducted through the Cochrane collaboration showed that antidepressants are effective for depression comorbid with a wide range of medical conditions and are generally well tolerated by patients with medical illness. There are some important considerations with the use of specific medications. For example, nortriptyline is effective in treating people with diabetes and depression but it has been found to worsen glucose control. The effect of psychotropic medication-related weight gain on insulin resistance is also an important issue to be considered. On the other hand, amitriptyline and dual-action antidepressants also play an important role in treating chronic painful physical conditions.

One important caution in using antidepressants in the medically ill group is the risk of adverse events related to safety issues of particular antidepressants, antidepressant side-effects and interactions with other drugs. Cautions about the use of antidepressants in the medically ill are listed as follows:

- Avoid antidepressants with potential safety concerns for interactions with the physical illness; e.g. tertiary amine TCAs in cardiac disease or bupropion in epilepsy.
- Avoid antidepressants with side-effects that may exacerbate the physical illness, e.g. nortriptyline in diabetes.
- Avoid antidepressants with potential drug interactions with other drugs used to treat the physical illness, e.g. nefazodone with quinidine.
- Start low, go slow and keep going, i.e. start with lower than usual doses of medications and titrate up slowly but continue to full therapeutic doses as needed.

Evidence-based treatment recommendations for treating depression in specific comorbid medical conditions are summarized in Table 13.3.

Bibliography

Addington D, Addington J, Maticka-Tyndale E, Joyce J. Reliability and validity of a depression rating scale for schizophrenics. *Schizophr Res* 1992; **6**: 201–8.

Enns M, Swenson JR, McIntyre RS *et al*. Clinical guidelines for the treatment of depressive disorders. VII. Comorbidity. *Can J Psychiatry* 2001; **46** (Suppl. 1): 79S–92S.

Gill D, Hatcher S. Antidepressants for depression in people with physical illness (Cochrane Review). *Cochrane Database Syst Rev* 2000; **4**: CD001312.

Table 13.3 Recommendations for MDD comorbid with Axis III (physical) disorders

Condition	Treatment choice	
	Psychotherapy	Pharmacotherapy
General medical disorders	Social support; psychotherapy (elderly) [Level 1]	Selective serotonin re-uptake inhibitors (SSRIs); novel antidepressants; tricyclic antidepressants (TCAs); psychostimulants [Level 1]
Cardiac disease	Cognitive behavioural therapy (CBT) [Level 3]	Fluoxetine; paroxetine; sertraline [Level 2] Nortriptyline [Level 2]
Cancer	No studies found	Fluoxetine; mianserin; paroxetine [Level 2] Amitriptyline; desipramine [Level 2]
Diabetes	Cognitive behavioural therapy (CBT) [Level 2]	Fluoxetine; sertraline [Level 2] Nortriptyline [Level 2] and other norepinephrine-acting TCAs may worsen glucose control, therefore not recommended
HIV/AIDS	Interpersonal psychotherapy (ITP); group social support; Cognitive behavioural therapy (CBT) [Level 2]	Fluoxetine [Level 1] Paroxetine; desipramine; imipramine [Level 2] Sertraline [Level 3]
Parkinson's disease	No studies found	Nortriptyline [Level 2] Paroxetine; sertraline [Level 3]
Stroke disease	CBT no more effective than placebo, therefore not recommended [Level 2]	Citalopram; fluoxetine; nortriptyline; sertraline [Level 1] Psychostimulants [Level 3]

Glassman AH, O'Connor CM, Califf RM *et al*. Sertraline treatment of major depression in patients with acute MI or unstable angina. *JAMA* 2002; **288** (6): 701–9.

Keller MB, McCullough JP, Klein DN *et al*. A comparison of nefazodone, the cognitive behavioral-analysis system of psychotherapy, and their combination for the treatment of chronic depression. *N Engl J Med* 2000; **342**: 1462–70.

Koerner K, Linehan MM. Research on dialectical behavior therapy for patients with borderline personality disorder. *Psychiatr Clin North Am* 2000; **23**: 151–67.

Krishnan KR, Delong M, Kraemer H *et al.* Comorbidity of depression with other medical diseases in the elderly. *Biol Psychiatry* 2002; **52**: 559–88.

Lesperance F, Frasure-Smith N. Depression in patients with cardiac disease: a practical review. *J Psychosom Res* 2000; **48**: 379–91.

Newport DJ, Nemeroff CB. Assessment and treatment of depression in the cancer patient. *J Psychosom Res* 1998; **45**: 215–37.

Rocca P, Marchiaro L, Cocuzza E, Bogetto F. Treatment of borderline personality disorder with risperidone. *J Clin Psychiatry* 2002; **63**: 241–4.

Zanarini MC, Frankenburg FR. Olanzapine treatment of female borderline personality disorder patients: a double-blind, placebo-controlled pilot study. *J Clin Psychiatry* 2001; **62**: 849–54.

Index